MW01167300

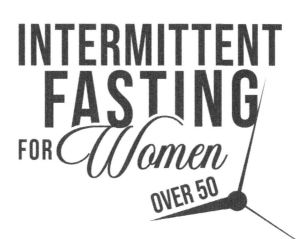

INTERMITTENT FASTING FOR Women OVER 50

Master the Secrets of Fasting to Promote Longevity by Losing Weight, Reset your Metabolism and Increase your Life Energy thanks to the Wonders of Metabolic Autophagy.

© Copyright 2021 - All rights reserved.

The content contained within this book may not be reproduced, duplicated or transmitted without direct writ- ten permission from the author or the publisher. Under no circumstances will any blame or legal responsibility be held against the publisher, or author, for any damages, reparation, or monetary loss due to the information contained within this book. Either directly or indirectly.

Legal Notice:

This book is copyright protected. This book is only for personal use. You cannot amend, distribute, sell, use, quote or paraphrase any part, or the content within this book, without the consent of the author or publisher.

Disclaimer Notice:

Please note the information contained within this document is for educational and entertainment purposes only. All effort has been executed to present accurate, up to date, and reliable, complete information. No warranties of any kind are declared or implied. Readers acknowledge that the author is not engaging in the rendering of legal, financial, medical or professional advice. The content within this book has been derived from various sources. Please consult a licensed professional before attempting any techniques outlined in this book. By reading this document, the reader agrees that under no circumstances is the author responsible for any losses, direct or indirect, which are incurred as a result of the use of information contained within this document, including, but not limited to, errors, omissions, or inaccuracies.

CONTENTS

INTRODUCTION

All our life we've been told to stay healthy, eat well, make some exercise. And we did it, in and out, some of us more than others.

Me, I was struggling to keep my weight off. The busy hours of work during the day and the keeping up with the house and the family during... any other moment, made my life too cluttered to follow any eat-better-get-better plan. Until I discovered that it's not much about *what* you eat, as much as *when* you eat it. I came to understand the wonders of planning the way I was feeding myself, of having a clear schedule for meals, and - more importantly - to respect it. It just took a pinch of willpower. From that moment on, life became shinier and merrier. I was feeling good.

I had found out the amazing power of Intermittent Fasting.

Women over 50 can benefit from intermittent fasting, especially when it comes to weight loss and, consequentially, longevity. It's really more straightforward than most people believe and it's also something that I feel like suggesting everyone I care about. Intermittent fasting may also help with some less known issues, like glucose intolerance, and is important for maintaining brain health as we age.

Before you know it, you've reached your fifties and are starting to notice changes in your anatomy. Grey stripes run through the hair, the skin is loose, and parts of the body aren't as supple as they once were. Fat forms and refuses to move, particularly around the belly button. Sounds familiar? It was to me.

Belly fat for once is a serious health issue that must be tackled. It becomes very difficult to lose any weight, let alone belly fat, after a woman reaches a certain age. It's part of our responsibility toward our body to act, and do it fast and relentlessly.

Intermittent fasting has been notoriously shown to help people lose weight, but it can also decrease the risk of cancer in middle-aged women by detoxing their organisms, along with other benefits like slowing the symptoms of ageing, increasing fertility, and reducing the risk of disease. It aids in the acceleration of the metabolism, the increase of energy and vitality, and let's not overlook the one that has been more fruitful for me: improving my confidence and self-esteem!

This book is a perfect read for all ladies, as we are going to shed light on and demistify how intermittent fasting can aid 360° our lives. Let's get started.

CHAPTER ONE

Getting to Know Intermittent Fasting

Lower metabolism, achy joints, decreased muscle mass, and sleep problems: some well known not-so-friendly companions of those who have kissed goodbyed their 50 for a while now. Simultaneously, losing weight, including the dangerous belly fat, is something that we all should strive for, and that will significantly lower the risk of major health problems including diabetes, heart attacks, and cancer. If we have passed 50 already and still have not taken preacautions, well, it's time to act. And one answer-them-all action can be intermittent fasting.

But what does intermittent fasting refer to exactly? The term fasting is familiar to almost all of us. The motives for fasting differ from one person to another, throughout the ages. It was (and still is) a religious ritual for some; they sacrificed meals in order to devote to prayer. People in the past would go out hunting or farming, to then only eat when resting. Others, unfortunately, have no reason other than they just don't have enough food.

Each of the above-mentioned fasting habits is not prolonged fasting. It is not a religious ritual, nor is it inspired by the absence of time or food - it is a preference. It's best characterised as an eating pattern that alternates between periods of eating and periods of fasting, each lasting a fixed amount of time. The 16:8

cycle, for example, includes a fasting time of 16 hours and an eating period of 8 hours.

The first historic appearance of intermittent fasting goes back to Hippocrates, the father of ancient medicine, over 2000 years ago. He strongly believed that the body had to be purified to be healed. He prepared his patients to medical treatments making them fast for long periods of time, and thousands of years later we still believe in this method, that has now Benn accepted and systemized.

Intermittent fasting is a type of time-restricting eating that requires eating food and stopping it (or fasting) for the rest of the day over, for example, an 8-hour window. It's the best way to optimize your daily meals so that you get the most out of them.

Giving the body more time to absorb food has been found to be more effective for weight loss than merely having a calorie deficit. The key principle in play in this diet is not to change the things you eat significantly, but the precise timing of consuming them.

The Science Of Intermittent Fasting

We burn calories at any given time, but according to experimental research relative to feeding times, we burn more fat during fasting periods. However, we burn calories at all times, and these calories come from fats and glucose (carbs) in various amounts. Insulin hormone is released via the pancreas to cope with the glucose molecules in the bloodstream when we eat food, particularly carbohydrates.

Glucose is either used to provide nutrition or processed as glycogen or fat. A higher percentage of calories will come from fat if you haven't eaten for a long time and the plasma glucose is low. Therefore, you're going to burn more calories. Fantastic as it sounds, these findings also indicate that when calories are equalised, intermittent fasting is not equivalent to other calorie-restrictive diets.

In fact we burn more fat during fasting periods than during eating periods, even while we're on particular calories restrictive diets.

If you haven't eaten in quite a long time and your blood glucose content is low, fat can make up a greater portion of your calories. Therefore, you're going to burn more of them.

This means that the success of intermittent fasting isn't dependent on the fact that you magically lose more fat during the fasting period. It results from physically aiding you in absorbing less calories. Let me illustrate why:

During the feeding window, if you ingest 2,000 calories and only burn 1,000 calories in this same window, the additional 1,000 calories will be processed for future consumption as fat and glycogen. You will burn more fats during your fasting time, but the fuel will come from your accumulated fat from your eating window. If you burn 2,000 calories during your fasting window, 1,000 will come from the food you ate before, and the remainder will come from body fat.

Intermittent fasting can help retain lean body mass during weight loss, while boosting insulin sensitivity.

INTERMITTENT FASTING:
A GENTLER ALTERNATIVE FOR WOMEN OVER 50

Many think that Intermediate fasting is just juice cleanses. It's not. I love juices, especially because adding what you're going to know later on as superfoods, you can make some explosive health bombs. But you can't live healthy just by drinking juices. Intermittent fasting, being one of the most common health and fitness phenomena in the world, is often misunderstood. It requires alternating fasting and feeding periods, and it is sustained by many trials that have found that it can help you lose weight, improve your metabolic health, shield you from disease, and maybe even help you live longer.

The point of Intermittent fasting is understanding when to do the "switch" between eating and fasting and the proportion in which you should practice one or the other. The food you consume is important but not as important in the fasting theory as when you should eat it. There are several distinct types of intermittent fasting, all of which break the day or week into feeding and fasting cycles. If you think about it, the majority of people already "fast" while sleeping every day. One of the ways to practice extended fasting is by progressively extending the fasting you are already doing. By missing breakfast and consuming your first lunch at noon you are already prompting your body to activate some of the beneficial effects of fasting. Easy? At first maybe not so much. But once using your will becomes a habit, you won't even notice. If then you also consume your last meal by 8 pm, you're technically fasting for 16 hours a day, which means feeding just within 8 hours per day. And you'd be already doing a 16/8 fasting, one of the most commonly used type of intermittent fasting. You can be a pro at this in no time.

INTERMITTENT FASTING:
A SAFE WAY TO BOOST METABOLISM

Let's focus on metabolism.

The mechanism by which your body produces and burns energy from food is referred to as metabolism. To breathe, think, absorb, pump blood, stay warm in the cold, and remain cool in the sun, you rely on your metabolism. It's a common myth that rising your metabolism will help you eat more calories and lose weight. Unfortunately, there are more metabolism-boosting misconceptions than successful methods. Several myths will backfire, for example "if you feel you are burning more calories than you really are, you can eat more than you should". In reality things you can't regulate, such as your age, sex, and genes, can determine whether your metabolism is quick or slow. Physical disfunction's as a slow thyroid can also reduce the metabolism.

Since our metabolism tends to slow down with age, we are prone to gain weight as we grow older, and we become less healthy.

Work and families take the toll as we neglect fitness. We lose muscle and add weight because we do not walk as much. We can also have an hard time controlling our meals as we grow older. When people grow older, their innate appetite control tends to fade. Big meals will easily add up if we are not careful.

Spacing your meals during the day could deter you from feeling too hungry and over-eat. Many athletes spend periods of their training time eating smaller quantities of food more often.

If you have a hard time controlling your appetite, three meals a day could be a good start and a safer choice rather than many small snacks to add up to a balanced intake. Listen to the appetite 's signs and feed while you're hungry, just enough. Of course limit high-sugar and high-fat snacks.

A very good practice is to maintain a food log to always have a trace of your daily intake and especially to hold you accountable for your daily eating choices.

Metabolism vs. Fat Burning

Many individuals loosely use the words metabolism and fat burning mixing them together. Even if they are related, these words do not mean the same thing. When talking about energy expenditure, is common practice to use the word "burning", although this is not entirely accurate. Fat burning is the mechanism by which your fat cells release energy packages, or fatty acid molecules, into the bloodstream. Your muscles then (but also your lungs, heart and other organs) break these fatty acids and use their energy for their activities. "Fat burning" turns a bunch of peanuts into a few running strides. An improved capacity to execute this fat burning process means you could eat more fat than what you were used to, but that doesn't actually mean your metabolism has picked up. If you were to go hungry, for example, your body would reduce your energy intake to save energy. If this is the case, the fat-to-energy process would augment, and there wouldn't actually be any other energy supply except fat and eventually some protein for your body to use. Your metabolism though will decrease. The "fat burning" job makes about 90% of your metabolism.

Those that wish to keep their body fat down and stay in shape should improve their energy intake by exercising and consuming a healthy diet, as well as increase the amount of fat burned with the correct way of fasting for you. This would lead to a drop in body fat as well as a progressively increased stamina for workouts.

INTERMITTENT FASTING:
EFFECT ON CELLS AND HORMONES

Although fasting for a prolonged period of time will reduce your metabolic rate, intermittent fasting has been shown to speed up the fasting process by around 14 percent.

But how does this translate in our body?

Several things happen in your body on a cellular and molecular basis as you fast. Your body hormone levels changes, for instance, to make retained body fat more available. Essential repair mechanisms and gene expression modifications are often triggered by your cells.

When you fast, your body undergoes the following changes:

• Human Growth Hormone (HGH): Growth hormone's levels skyrocket, rising as much as 5-fold. This results in fat loss and muscle gain benefits.

• Insulin: Insuline Immunity increases while insulin levels decrease significantly. Higher insulin levels improve the usability of retained body fat.

• Cellular Repair: As you fast, your cells tend to repair themselves. Autophagy is a mechanism in which cells digest and destroy old and damaged proteins that have collected within them, providing more energy.

• Gene Expression: variations in gene regulation related to survival and disease prevention are promoted by a correct fasting period.

The health effects of intermittent fasting are responsible for these variations in hormone levels, cell structure and gene expression.

IMPROVING LONGEVITY

Intermittent fasting has been found to disrupt the mechanisms and progression of those body conditions that can lead to death, meaning that those that perform intermittent fasting have a healthy and longer life on a daily basis compared to those who consume three meals a day or just reduce calories intake. This way of fasting encourages our bodies to rebuild weakened tissues while also replacing stressed out and aged tissues, resulting in anti-aging effects that allow both organs and cells to function properly.

Intermittent fasting's regenerative capacity of the immune system promotes the development and increases the number of white blood cells (WBCs, or leukocytes), which are the predominant defense in which our body battles infections. In this way Intermittent fasting helps our body to purge old and weakened cells and replace them with more effective immune system cells. According to a study, a 72-hour fasting is suitable to assist cancer patients to encounter less side effects during chemotherapeutic administrations, which are known to cause significant immune system harm. While more tests are necessary to confirm this assertion, several researchers have suggested that intermittent fasting is very useful for those patients and seniors who are immunosuppressed.

Talking about skin's longevity, intermittent fasting also rejuvenates the skin. As patients suffering from acne are aware, the safest way to manage the acne disturb is to eat unprocessed foods and decrease the ingestion of dairy products via our diets.

One of the major causes of any kind of inflammatory disorders is food sensitivities. Following your fasting periods, remember to eat food one item at a time, and monitor any changes in your skin tone to decide which foods are best for you and which one you should avoid.

Being a diet that favors protein food, Intermittent fasting also has positive consequences for our hair and nails, allowing them to grow stronger and healthier.

INTERMITTENT FASTING: **ENHANCING SPIRITUAL WELLBEING**

This is one of those topics which is never mentioned when talking bout any kind of fasting, but which I find of the utmost importance.

As we've seen above, fasting has been practiced since humankind inception. It's an archetypical image and memory engraved in our minds.

We shouldn't underestimate the importance of our inner well being and connection with the spiritual, being it God or whatever we believe in, included ourself.

I believe that Intermittent fasting, combined with a balanced lifestyle, leads to a stronger sense of faith. During their fasting times, practitioners have affirmed a general sense of tranquility. In addition fasting can help control mood through stress management and reduction of anxiety. And what could even sound more surprising is that fasting is sometimes also prescribed as a natural solution for a variety of sexual and mental issues.

Experts agree that our cognition is embodied, meaning our body is a reflection of what's going on inside our mind. So if you're into meditation, that is something that goes very well with the practice of reprogramming your eating cycles. Committing to some inner work helps us focus on losing weight without avoiding the emotional and mental being that we are, understanding why the weight is showing up in the first place. Whether you are fasting for spiritual purposes or not, intermittent fasting will strengthen your interaction with nature and the rest of the world. You'll get a more optimistic attitude and a clearer mind in general.

CHAPTER TWO

Intermittent Fasting: How Does It Work?

To comprehend how intermittent fasting contributes to fat loss, we must first comprehend the distinction between the fed and fasted states.

When the body digests and consumes food, it is in a fed state. Usually, after you start feeding, the fed state begins and continues for 3 to 5 hours as the body digests and consumes the food you just ate. Since your insulin levels are elevated while you're in the fed state, it's tough for your body to burn fat.

During that time frame, the body reaches a state known as the post-absorptive state, which is a fancy way of suggesting that it isn't consuming the food. After the last meal, the post-absorptive state continues for 8 to 12 hours, which is when you reach the fasting state. Since your insulin levels are low, it is much easier for your body to lose fat in a fasting state.

Your body will burn fat that has been unavailable during the fed state while you are in the fasting state.

Because we do not reach the fasting period until 12 hours after our last meal, it is unusual for our bodies to be in this state of fat burning. This is one of the reasons why, without adjusting what they eat, how often they eat, or how much they exercise, many people who begin intermittent fasting will lose weight. Fasting causes a fat-burning state in your body that you seldom achieve on a daily feeding schedule.

An eating plan that varies between fasting and eating on a daily basis is intermittent fasting. We've been saying that Intermittent fasting has been shown to help people lose weight and avoid or even cure illness. So how do you go about doing it? And is it secure?

The Role of Sugar

Intermittent fasting can be achieved in a number of ways, but they all revolve around choosing daily food and fasting hours. For example, every day, you can try to eat only during an eight-hour cycle and fast for the rest of the day. Alternatively, you might opt to eat just one meal a day, two days a week. There are several intermittent fasting schedules that differ for eat/fasting proportion. A great role in deciding which kind of fasting approach is played by sugar.

The depletion of liver glycogen stores (sugars) leads to the production of ketones from fatty acids[1]. After a period of time without sugar, the body's sugar reserves are drained, the fat takes the place of the sugar and is consumed instead. This is referred as metabolic switching.

----

[1] https://www.nature.com/articles/nrn.2017.156

"For most Americans, who feed in their waking hours, prolonged fasting compares with the usual feeding schedule," says Mark Mattson, during his appearance at TEDx talk. "If someone eats three meals a day, with snacks, and they don't workout, then they run on those calories every time they feed, not burning their fat stocks."

By prolonging the time after your body has eaten all the calories ingested during the last meal, intermittent fasting goes into action, begins to burn fat starting to be effective.

The Key Role of Insulin

Our bodies can run on two kin of fuel: glucose and fat. We get glucose from carbs and proteins present in our meals. Fat comes from meat, fish, certain kind of fruit, eggs, oils, etc.). We can run on both fuels, but we can't make use of them at the same time. When we go through calorie restrictions we try to push our body to switch from glucose fuel to fat fuel. The process of burning fat instead of glucose is called ketosis. For ketosis to happen we must stop any glucose intake, for our insulin hormone to work in the way we want.

Insulin is a fundamental hormone with several critical functions, and it's worth to focus a bit more on the explanation of the mechanism behind it. The main two activities that are of great interest to us are that it facilitate the cells' glucose absorption and assist with the fat storage functions. It's important to keep the sensitivity of our organism to insulin because if it becomes resistant to it these functions can get disrupted. With lowered sensitivity our cells respond lowly to insulin signals, and as a consequence the level of sugar in your blood stay to an unnecessary and dangerous high level. As the sugar needs to be lowered, our pancreas creates more insulin which leads to an overloading of insulin, more than what our cells could cope with, as the amount of sugar remains too high. The cells cannot accept any other sugar so insulin has no other option than converting the sugar in excess in fat. This is why as long as there is a lot of sugar around our blood, our organism remains in a fat-storage mode.

One way to solve this situation is to restrict the sugar intake restricting the calories that we introduce into our organism. It takes 8 to 12 hours for the insulin level to sink to acceptable levels. That is why intermittent fasting can help us to battle insulin resistance.

Until the insulin level has not reached an acceptable level, we are going to store fat. This means that after a meal our bodies take 8 to 12 hours to normalize the insulin level: if we eat anything within this range (before 8 hours) the insulin level would spike up and our bodies would stop burning fat. You can see how unluckily it is to get into a fat-burning state in normal conditions, when our body is fed frequently and is not enduring physical effort. Our wrong habits are responsible for insulin resistance and ultimately one of the most dangerous issue in our society, which is the large spread of obesity.

INTERMITTENT FASTING: **LET'S GET STARTED**

Intermittent fasting is a way of feeding, not a diet. It's a form of preparing your meals so that you get the best bang for your buck.

Most significantly, it's a perfect way to get lean without seriously reducing your calorie intake. Actually, most of the time, when you begin intermittent fasting, you'll try to keep your calories the same.

With all that said, losing weight is the biggest reason people pursue intermittent fasting.

Intermittent fasting is anyway also a healthy way to retain muscle strength when gaining weight, as many athletes know.

Since it needs relatively little behaviour adjustment, intermittent fasting is one of the best methods we have for gaining weight while retaining a healthier weight, when a high protein intake is combined with focused exercise. This is a really positive aspect for those extra sporty people whose main goal is not be lighter on the scale, but completely control their musclular mass. This confirms that intermittent fasting falls under the category of those things "easy enough for you to really do it, but important enough to make a difference".

USE THE RIGHT MINDSET

Adjust your mindset, then your food habits, and eventually your life. The right mindset is crucial if you want to succeed in fasting and make your life better. To achieve my results in a definitive way I had to go through a learning curve to control my will, and it paid its dividend. So I want you to learn how to master your best mentality.

Why is your success crucial?

Mindset is the single most significant thing that affects a person's performance. What you consistently think about has a direct effect on your conduct and not the other way around. So, getting this basic ingredient right is a necessary condition to undergo with the right mind-tools your journey in fasting. Mindset, a relatively vaporous factor that makes a major difference, is the main dividing factor between those who excel and those who do not. And you must learn to master yours if you are serious about finding success in every aspect of your life.

Here are six key reasons why.

1. Developing a Healthy Self-esteem

To accomplish something worthwhile, you must first assume you are worthy of doing so. It makes no sense what people say on the outside. The internal debate, the words that tell how we view and measure our worth, whether positively or negatively, are the foundations of self-esteem. Our self-concept is framed within the comprehensive view we have about ourselves.

A good and optimistic mindset is important for the production of healthy self-esteem. It's a powerful instrument that shapes our everyday self-talk and strengthens our most personal self-perceptions, behaviours, and emotions. So, become the gatekeeper of positivity and motivation in your mind and plant seeds rather than criticism and doubt.

You have to be able to support yourself and believe in your strengths in order to do something amazing. Success is what you make, not something that just happens. You must be self-assured enough to ignore the derogatory voices in your mind. Don't give up on the things you believe in—and, most importantly, don't give up on yourself.

2. Formulating A Winning Perspective

There are few qualities more important than perspective when it comes to performance. If we perceive our glass as half full or half empty has a significant impact on how we want to apply value to circumstances and situations. The reality is that perspective is everything when it comes to attitude. The way we perceive knowledge and interpret the world around us is naturally influenced by our foundational values, perceptions and prejudices. Getting a good outlook improves the odds of creating a winning plan and achieving long-term results.

3. Harnessing Drive

The unwavering determination to accomplish a significant aim is known as motivation. It requires the process of building a vision for accomplishment and investing in a well planned effort over time. It would be impossible, at best, to accomplish most targets without drive.

This involves a certain mentality. It can quickly urge someone to question the status quo and step beyond comfort zones with the ability to direct attention and foster dedication to a greater cause. People who have ambition are self-motivated and still seek to do more. They don't waste time moaning about their circumstances; instead, they work hard to change them.

Knowing what you desire and being able to work hard to accomplish it are two entirely different things. Knowing what you want to do motivates you. It doesn't not change you if it doesn't challenge you. Set high expectations and don't rest until you've achieved them.

4. Facing Adversity

The road to your achievement is expected to contain some degree of adversity, no matter what purpose you aim to accomplish. However, you will need to grow strong skin and learn to tackle each obstacle head-on if you want to get through the rough patches.

This is where attitude plays a vital part. Adversity is measuring the mettle of one to the heart. An individual may feel justified in succumbing to defeat after facing severe hardship. It can feel like an easy path for them. Yet, a true testament to the strength of a robust mentality is the ability to step through the flames, get knocked down and not knocked out.

You're going to get easy sailing all the way to your destination – you'll have to tackle hurdles and difficulties, and you'll have to find a way to overcome difficulty in the end. Many individuals surrender to the obstacles they face because it feels like the simpler way out. However, you would be more likely to continue battling and overcome future challenges once you have the right frame of mind.

5. Achieving The Underlying Goal

Goal-setting is a multi-faceted process, with the most visible measure of progress being accomplishment. However, you could not get that far if you don't have the right attitude. An endeavour that easily eludes even the most well-intentioned people needs more than a simple lukewarm motivation to excel in achieving an aim.

The rubber hits the road when it comes to attitude. Internal resilience, taken a little further, is what defines when anyone can dig deep and persevere in the face of difficulty in order to excel, or ultimately give up. It entails exercising confidence, maintaining effort over long stretches, and using self-talk to progress beyond each crucial step until the fundamental objective is eventually accomplished.

By giving more serious attention to your attitude, both of the above becomes more realistic. It is bound to boost the general state of your self-esteem, drive, inspiration, and capacity to conquer challenges you are likely to face along the way to get yourself into the right mindset.

6. Your State of Mind Can Change Your Perspective on Things

Getting a pessimistic outlook will deter you from viewing it from the right angle. You'll be more able to notice the negative sides of your condition and the challenges that will hinder you from achieving your target. Maintaining a constructive frame of mind, though, will help you properly assess the conditions and maintain a more proactive attitude.

Furthermore, deciding to be optimistic and having a positive outlook would have a huge effect on your life. It will go a long way if you concentrate on positivity. Maintain a proactive mentality rather than a passive one. Give yourself reasons why you should and permission to go for it, instead of giving yourself reasons why you can't or shouldn't. Happiness never arrives from outside situations, but rather from inside. The value of an optimistic attitude appears to be overlooked by failed individuals, and this is one of the reasons that their goals often seem to be unachievable or the earliest challenge puts them away from achieving their goals. You're doing it for yourself, be happy about it!

Mindset Around Fasting

When it comes to your overall success and ability to reach your goals, managing hunger and sticking to your diet is vital. Intermittent fasting can help you achieve this, but while some people can fast for long periods of time with little difficulty, others, especially when first starting out, may find it more difficult.

Using the right mindset is merely another dietary setup that, when used correctly and in accordance with one's lifestyle, can be very effective for some people. It's important to keep this in mind when using intermittent fasting and know that, yes, it can bring incredible results, but these results are dependent on the achievement of 3 elements:

• Hitting your calorie and macronutrient goal

• Training consistently

• Applying progressive overload

This is valid with all diets, but if you're doing intermittent fasting or anything else, keep this in mind. Here are three techniques to help you embrace this mindset:

1. Base your objectives on realistic expectations of what is actually possible rather than what you wish was possible.

2. In your efforts, be single-minded and understand that the best path to success is consistent effort towards a singular goal.

3. Be patient and understand that just as you didn't lose your dream body in a day, week, or month, you won't be able to reclaim it in the same time frame.

If you insist in starving yourself after a binge, it's very unlikely you will ever carry out a proper fasting. Food and its restriction are not intended to be a reward or punishment for our bodies. When we remove the emotions from food, it becomes merely a means of fueling our bodies so that they can function to their full potential. We're more likely to make better choices in the kitchen when we're looking for those macro- and micronutrients in every meal. The same mindset needs to be held by fasting.

It's important to remember why you're intermittent fasting when you're doing it. This is not the moment to cut calories; our calorie targets will always be reached in a shortened meal timeframe rather than eating less calories in total. To help your body prevent insulin resistance, you might be involved in a 24-hour fasting or sporadic fasting because it runs in your family. You may be fasting after a few intense workouts and relying on hydration to help the body heal itself. Write down whatever the "why" is and keep it ready while you're fasting.

It's time to make a decision after you've found out why you're doing it. This decision involves not only consuming a nutritious meal the night before, but also clearing your mind. There will be difficult moments, especially the first days, but you will set yourself up for success by learning how you will resolve these moments before they happen! If you find yourself trying to cave in, are you looking for water or herbal tea? Are you going to call your accountability partner? Can you go on a stroll?

Fasting is extremely beneficial, and I am confident that you will be successful if you approach it with the right mindset. Remember, it's all in your mind.

CHAPTER THREE

Things You Should Know Before You Try Intermittent Fasting

Intermittent fasting doens't follow the shooting star pattern of your usual fad diet. It's more like a way of living that's been around for a very long time and is now an integral part of many cultures.

Before starting your journey though there are some side-effects that you should be aware of. Intermittent fasting, as every other diets, has some drawbacks and is not advised for all. Fasting over long periods of time and modifying one's eating routine may be dangerous to expectant mothers, people with diabetes, and those with eating disorders. It is important for pregnant women and diabetic patients to feed at frequent intervals. It's likely that not feeding for 16 hours could be detrimental to their well being. In such a scenario, please contact your nutritionist before attempting fasting.

. You Must Eat Healthy During the Feeding Period

Intermittent fasting does not exclude any category of foods, but it also does not encourage you to overindulge or drink unhealthy foods. You will only be able to see desired results by consuming nutritious meals in your feeding window and avoiding the consumption of unnecessary calories in the eating periods of the day.

. Fasting can be stopped at all times, whenever you have higher calorie needs.

When you are at risk of an eating disorder, you should stop fasting entirely. Intermittent fasting is strongly correlated with bulimia nervosa, and, as a result, there can be no diet associated with fasting for people who are vulnerable to an eating disorder. Having a family member with an eating disorder, perfectionism, impulsivity and mood disturbance are risk factors for an eating disorder.

. Do not get Dehydrated.

Don't hesitate to use your fasting window for drinking water. In most cases, it has been found that when fasting, people fail to drink water. Pay close attention to your hydration, a lack of water in out body can trigger headaches, difficulty in concentrating, and hunger. In each fasting window you should have water, unsweetened coffee or tea with 2 teaspoons of milk or diluted apple cider vinegar.

Since you will be eating no calories for lengthy stretches of time during the day, it is important that you remain hydrated to ensure that your body works correctly internally. When you're fasting, it's easy to ignore the fact that your body needs water to stay healthy.

Often, when you think you're starving, you're actually dehydrated instead. Just drink a glass of water next time you experience hunger pangs during your fasting window. It could easily make the sensation of hunger vanish.

. Do not fast for a prolonged period of time.

Opinions disagree on which intermittent fasting diet is better, but the scientific consensus agrees on one thing: you can lose weight if you consume more calories than you eat. Fasting can help you big time but very prolonged time while fasting can only be advised by a doctor or professional nutritionist.

. Take it slow.

You don't have to do 18 hours of fasting straight out from the gates. Give time for your body to adapt to your new eating habits. Those that hurry into action are going to have a more difficult time getting used to intermittent fasting.

Take it gently at first. For the first two weeks, begin by fasting for 12 hours. Increase your fasting hours to 14, 16, and so on as you get more relaxed. Do this before you obtain a form of fasting that you are satisfied with.

It needs time to get used to intermittent fasting. And time is also the element that'll make adhering to the diet soft and easy. You have the chance to tweak and change your eating routine to make it work into your lifestyle, because it is not a sudden change in your eating habits.

. Make it work on your own schedule.

Intermittent fasting can be easy, if you make it easy. The key is making your schedule fitting around it. Most of the people who have trouble making intermittent fasting work are those who try to adapt their day to the timetable of someone else. To make this work, you must strategically schedule *your* day to make the best out of your fasting hours.

Most of us operate on a daily 9-5. Others work late into the night or just half a day. Each of us have different commitments in our everyday lives, so you can't just copy someone else's schedule and expect it to work for you. By changing the fasting hours to match your own timetable you will find a stability that will make intermittent fasting much easier to manage.

A smart tip is to fast for the majority of the time while you're sleeping. So try to get as much sleep as possible, because hunger pangs are less likely to strike while you're asleep. You'll just have to wait a few hours after you wake up to break your fast.

Types Of Intermittent Fasting

As a way to potentially reduce weight, stave off disease, and maximise lifespan, this diet technique is increasing in popularity. However, depending on your lifestyle and priorities, you have many choices.

5:2 Fasting

This is one of the most commonly used, and most popular, Intermittent Fasting strategies. The execution of this kind of fasting involves eating regularly for 5 days, and then eat 500 or 600 calories a day for women and men, respectively, for the remaining two days.

The idea is that short fasting bursts keep you compliant. Should you be struggling on your fast days you know that soon will come a day with normal meals. Always bear to mind though that a 5:2 plan will work only if during the whole week we will stay on the lower calories side, rather than binging whatever we see around the kitchen.

Some bring this diet to the extreme with a zero calories consumption on the fasting days, but I think that is too much. The 5:2 approach focuses on restricting the calories and 500 a day for two days a week, is a sufficient and healthy way of doing it. Throughout the other five days of the week you follow a safe and normal diet. This technique typically involves a 300-calorie meal together with a 200-calorie meal on fasting days. When fasting, it's important to concentrate on high-fiber and high-protein foods to help fill you up while keeping calories down.

Why it works: By relying on just two days of calorie reduction, you put yourself in a spot to lose weight while still getting more comfortable when you get to eat something on those two days.

The catch: Well, the first time you try to adjust your eating habits you'll cut your calories a lot, which will take some planning and some deep breaths. It may not be easy at first, but hey, who wants it easy? On top of that, you do have to eat healthy on the other five days. I would advise against eating pizza and burgers for five days and lettuce and lemon wedges the next two.

DAY 1	DAY 2	DAY 3	DAY 4	DAY 5	DAY 6	DAY 7
Eats normally	Women: 500 calories Men: 600 calories	Eats normally	Eats normally	Women: 500 calories Men: 600 calories	Eats normally	Eats normally

16:8 Intermittent fasting

Probably the most common form of intermittent fasting today is the 16:8 technique. It is also called time-restricted fasting: you fast for 16 hours and restrict your eating window to 8 hours during the day. There are few variants that alter the window for eating to 7 or even 6 hours, which are to employ especially when you want to approach and prepare to the most demanding types of dietary regimens.

As you can imagine this is one of the easiest kind of fasting and also the one I advise to try as your first introduction to fasting. In fact most people miss breakfast as part of the 16-hour window. So, for example, you could eat between 12 and 8 p.m, making it a kind of regular day. However it is implicit that we should really avoid to eat junk food in between our two meals, even if that is within our eating window.

As an alternative one can opt to miss dinner instead. You could set your eating window between 9 am and 5 pm per day, if you fancy going to bed early and your stomach growling do not prevent you from sleeping.

This method of intermittent fasting, according to studies, will help you lose weight and likely even lower your cholesterol levels.

This simple method works because obviously you eat less calories when you are not eating as much as you are used to. Plus, the 16-hour fasting covers your sleeping hours, so unless you dream about eating, 7 or 8 hours of you 16 are going to pass effortlessly. Your body is working for you while you sleep! If you can do it you could even think about extending your sleeping time to get you closer to your eating window.

Changing your eating habits may be tough but this kind of fasting process is easy and flexible enough for you to start your journey with the right foot.

	DAY 1	DAY 2	DAY 3	DAY 4	DAY 5	DAY 6	DAY 7
Midnight 4 AM 8 AM	FAST	FAST	FAST	FAST	FAST	FAST	FAST
12 PM	First meal	First meal	First meal	First meal	First meal	First meal	First meal
4 PM	Last meal by 8pm	Last meal by 8pm	Last meal by 8pm	Last meal by 8pm	Last meal by 8pm	Last meal by 8pm	Last meal by 8pm
8 PM Midnight	FAST	FAST	FAST	FAST	FAST	FAST	FAST

One Meal A Day

One of the most extreme fasting methods, the OMAD (one meal a day) diet requires you to eat - as per its name - only one meal a day, for just one hour, which means fasting for the other 23 hours. This is an intense form of intermittent fasting, and as such it is not advised as your introductory step into the fasting practice.

A softer way to approach this diet is to have a normal meal (many prefer an evening or late afternoon meal) accompanied by 2 very light snacks distanced by 2 hours after or before your daily meal.

The calorie deficit leads to a weight loss but it may also assist in the reduction of some cardiovascular disease risk factors. However, being it the most hardcore type of fasting it is normal to feel the pangs of hunger so one of the most critical point to keep under control is to not let your craving lead to overeating during your meal.

If you do a great amount of exercises and training in your days, this is probably not the dietitian regimen I would suggest you, but if you're looking for a kind of fasting that brings results quick and your willing to extend it for short periods it is definitely a kind of intermittent fasting you should consider.

Last thing, to not overlook, is that if you develop a periodical habit to the OMAD, you would have found a solid way to improve your discipline and willpower, meaning that you're already one step closer not only to be a better version of you, but to everything you desire in life. Discipline is a muscle and it takes some sweat to develop, but if you're able to pull this off the psychological reward of accomplishment is going to be worth the effort.

Alternate-Day Fasting

As the name suggests, this diet entails fasting every other day. Eat-fast, eat-fast and so on. There are several different variations of this pattern, but generally it allows around 500 calories on fasting days. If you decide to go for this diet, you can play around with the calories intake, or pushing it near to zero when you feel comfortable with it.

The method had been popularised by Krista Varady, PhD, a nutrition professor at the University of Illinois in Chicago. According to this plan fasters are allowed to 25% of their daily calorie requirements (which are approximately 500 calories), while and nonfasting days can be regular eating days. This is a very common weight-loss technique. Dr. Varady and colleagues observed in a small study published in Nutrition Journal that alternate-day fasting was successful in helping obese adults lose weight. By week two, the side effects (such as hunger) diminished and the participants continued to become more comfortable with the diet by week four.

The calories on fasting days must be consumed with one meal of your preference, lunch or dinner.

A useful help for achieving results with this dietary regimen is constituted by fluids: drink a lot of water, tea (or herbal tea) and unsweetened coffee.

DAY 1	DAY 2	DAY 3	DAY 4	DAY 5	DAY 6	DAY 7
Eats normally	24-hour fast OR Eat only a few hundred calories	Eats normally	24-hour fast OR Eat only a few hundred calories	Eats normally	24-hour fast OR Eat only a few hundred calories	Eats normally

Eat-Stop-Eat Diet

This type of fasting calls for fasting once or twice a week, in a complete 24-hour fast. You might, for example, eat dinner at 6 p.m. and then fast until 6 p.m. of the following day. If you want to fast for more than one day a week one, make the two days of fasting not consecutive. If you are fairly consistent on the long run it's likely for this regimen to result in weight loss because of the total amount of calorie restriction.

In the days of the week in which you do not fast, you r allowed t heat normally, but once again, this means following a healthy regular eating schedule and not binging as an answer to a quick feeding desire fulfillment.

If you want to add some (fairly serious) exercise in order to boost the weight loss benefit, I suggest you to increase by 20% the calories intake the other nonfasting days. Adding exercise (and yoga!) is also a way to make the process simpler and more manageable while you are having a calorie deficit.

Also during this diet you may control hunger during fasting days drinking water, tea or coffee. This is the perfect fasting method for those who want to put together the fasting effort in just one of two days and then forget about it. I suggest getting on this fasting with 2 days a week.

DAY 1	DAY 2	DAY 3	DAY 4	DAY 5	DAY 6	DAY 7
Eats normally	24-hour fast	Eats normally	Eats normally	24-hour fast	Eats normally	Eats normally

Time-Restricted Fasting

This kind of fasting is also referred as "time-restricted eating".

See it like an introductory road to heavier forms of fasting. It simply requires you to choose an eating window the will need to be respected each day. The typical eating window ranges from 6 to 12 hours a day. As the most attentive would have noticed this is just a more flexible 16:8 fasting program. Maybe you would be more comfortable with a 12 hour fasting which is very similar to a regular day eating cycle. What changes here though is your mindset: too easy? Great! Do it in the right way then, eat only healthy food without snacking around. This program is an excellent way to "rest" in between different fasting methods or fasting periods.

Also this kind of fasting encourages authophagy and general health. You would be surprised about how many benefits your body will register just by sticking to your guns and show yourself discipline in peaceful times.

For example, set your meal window from 9 a.m. to 6 p.m. and be consistent to respect this window. This works really nicely with those of us who are very busy tending to our families or taking care of the house and have follow a fixed routine. Lay down your simple plan and be consisitent!

Whole-Day Fasting

This kind of fasting requires you to eat everyday but only once. Some people prefer to eat dinner and then nothing else until the following day's dinner. That brings the fasting time to 24 hours, dinner to dinner or lunch to lunch, which is the one I would suggest you and that definitely worked the best for me.

Until you're not completely used to get all of of your calories from one meal (and I'm also talking from a mentality standpoint) it may be difficult for your body to operate optimally.

The main challenges you may be facing is around dinner time, our body could get really hungry and that could drive you to consume not-so-great, calorie-dense aliments. Think about it: You're not exactly craving broccoli while you're ravenous. Once again tea, maybe flavored, or coffee can come to aid, but pay attention to not drink too much caffeine which can have harmful effects on your sleep, and if you're not sleeping, you can find yourself brain fog ged during the day, which will make fasting more difficult.

Overnight Fasting

When we come to a 12 hours fasting and a 12 hours period we talk about overnight fasting. One of the easiest way to fasting, but simplicity is key to anything done well. For instance you can choose to avoid feeding after dinner, say 7 pm, and start eating only after 7 am the next morning. At the 12-hour mark, autophagy will still come into play, but with milder cellular advantages.

This is the minimum number of hours advised for fasting, but this approach has the bonus of being quick to execute and requires the lead amount of will power. For the most part, you don't have to miss meals; what you do, if anything, is eliminate a snack at bedtime. However, this approach does not completely harness the benefits of fasting. If you're fasting to lose weight, a narrower fasting window ensures you'll have the full benefits on your weight and general health. Use this just as dipping your toe and entering in the correct mind state of fasting. Use this as a launch pad to take off with one to the other fasting types.

The Warrior Diet

With the bulk of feeding occurring during the night, this diet is much different from the others. Ori Hofmekler, a fitness blogger, coined the word "Warrior Diet." This diet entails consuming only small amounts of fresh fruits and vegetables, diary products and hard-boiled eggs during the day, then eating within a 4-hour eating span in one big meal at night, or in the afternoon. The most curious trait of this diet is that during those 4 hours, even for those who choose to have them at night, you can eat - and actually invited to overeat - any kind of food that you want.

With such original claims it's no wonder this approach has not yet sufficient scientific data to back it up. But even though there is no clear study on the Warrior Diet, it is a diet which is getting more and more popular, with its giving room for some food during its fasting window. Even if a bit impractical, given the requirement of eating at night, its popularity is rising especially among gym lovers. The period in which you are allowed to greater amount of food is reduced; during this period the diet makes large use of paleo foods. Being the fasting time a 20 hours period it is stricter than other types of intermittent fasting.

	DAY 1	DAY 2	DAY 3	DAY 4	DAY 5	DAY 6	DAY 7
Midnight							
4 AM	Eating only small amounts of vegetables and fruits	Eating only small amounts of vegetables and fruits	Eating only small amounts of vegetables and fruits	Eating only small amounts of vegetables and fruits	Eating only small amounts of vegetables and fruits	Eating only small amounts of vegetables and fruits	Eating only small amounts of vegetables and fruits
8 AM							
12 PM							
4 PM	Large meal	Large meal	Large meal	Large meal	Large meal	Large meal	Large meal
8 PM							
Midnight							

This diet, like other intermittent fasting strategies, can lead to weight loss when a caloric deficit is reached.

Juice Fasting

This plan involves the consumption of five juices and one broth during the day. You can select and choose which juice recipes you want to try based on your tastes. I suggest you to try many but to stick to a core of four or five ingredients and rotate them if you want to keep the shopping to a minimum. Be sure that the consumption of vegetables is at least equal to the intake of fruit, however. The morning juices in this plan are supposed to be a little sweeter, whilst the afternoon juices are more vegetable-based. In the evenings, the warm juice is made to taste as much like pudding as possible!

The plan has a five day schedule; after a couple of days, however, feel free to stop and gauge how your organism is reacting. Juice fasting is usually mostly pulled off as part of a detox vacation where yoga, walks and spas are involved. In other words, not amid everyday life's hustle and bustle, as it would give you enough energy to go through them efficiently. As a result, most people tend to have a juice cleanse during the weekends. You can drink juices throughout the day at frequent intervals rather than sipping them during the whole day.

Skipped Meals

Lastly we have what is the most casual form of fasting, so casual that even the word fasting may sound too much. It's the little brother of fasting: when your body doesn't require to be fed, do not eat. It's "just" about listening to our own organism. Sometimes we are hungry, sometimes we think we are hungry but we're actually not, it's just habit to eat. The premise is that you can miss some meals (1 to 3) when you do not feel the necessity to eat, or when you are too busy to do it. This way you are naturally lowering calories and as a consequence you are a bit closer to your weight goal.

In this case, weight loss may be slower, but when you chose which meals you want to miss, you are in control. But control also means that you'll need to make deliberate efforts to miss a meal. This can be difficult for us because we are used to feed at precise hours of the day, and when that time comes most of us feed immediately.

Whatever type of intermittent fasting you're going to choose, bear in mind that calories and food consistency are always vital and

DAY 1	DAY 2	DAY 3	DAY 4	DAY 5	DAY 6	DAY 7
Breakfast	Skipped Meal	Breakfast	Breakfast	Breakfast	Breakfast	Breakfast
Lunch	Lunch	Lunch	Lunch	Lunch	Lunch	Lunch
Dinner	Dinner	Dinner	Dinner	Skipped Meal	Dinner	Dinner

should not be forgotten. Sometimes, when they utilise intermittent fasting as a protective net, individuals may side-line food consistency or over indulge in calories. This will not result to be successful in the long term, and your health will be compromised.

When practising intermittent fasting, consuming a safe, well-balanced diet is important. If in your non-fasting days you consume junk food and extra calories you can't hope to lose weight. The quality of your food must be up to par with the control on your own body.

Ease Your Way Into Fasting Plan

I know it may seem daunting at first but there is an easier way to get into an intermittent fasting diet. I will give you a strategy to get into one of the most famous meal plans we have talked about, the 16:8.

This strategy allows you to proceed step by step since you are extending day after day the hours in which you fast.

DAY 1

Goal: 12 h Fast I 12 h Eat

Start by fasting only 12 hours on your first day. From here add one additional hour each day. This way it is easier for your brain and body to get used to the new way of feeding.

DAY 2

Goal: 13 h Fast I 11 h Eat

Today you will be increasing your fast to 13 hours. It's only 60 minutes more, which is quite doable, isn't it? You can start to consume more whole food and start avoiding sugar and processed food.

DAY 3

<u>Goal</u>: 14 h Fast I 10 h Eat

You have now reached the 14 hours fasting day. Once you passed this step, you have proved yourself that you can do it. You need to start rewarding yourself and send your brain some positive signals: we're a great team, together we can do it!

DAY 4

<u>Goal</u>: 15 h Fast I 9 h Eat

Fasting 15 hours will make you one step closer to your goal, and you're only on your fourth day. Make sure to fill up the tank with a high protein lunch to support your weight-loss intentions.

DAY 5

<u>Goal</u>: 16 h Fast I 8 h Eat

Congratulations! You have reached your goal: 16 hours of fasting, and it has been easier than you expected. Now you have to stay strong and allow your body to get used to this new dietary regimen. When experiencing hunger, I suggest you drink a cup of black coffee, this might help you both mentally and physically . Coffee is an appetite-suppressing beverage abundant in antioxidants. Just don't exaggerate. If you're not into coffee a green tea will work too since it contains caffeine.

DAY 6

Goal: 16 h Fast I 8 h Eat

While maintaining the 16 hours fasting, begin to insert some light exercise in your routine. Start with a 20-minute walk, preferably outside. This will also improve your mood and will switch your focus from hunger. Listen to music or a podcast (or this book in audiobook format!).

DAY 7

Goal: 16 h Fast I 8 h Eat

You made it! Think about the accomplishment you achieved and congratulate yourself. Take picture of your body and start taking notes about your progress: record your weight, write down the sensations, the reaction of your body, and the improvements you have made.

Continue with the 16 hours fasting for another week, write down how your body reacts and gets better.

As the weeks go by, notice every change in your body and in your self-image.

Intermittent Fasting Exercises

If you've ever gone on a restricting diet for an extended amount of time, you know how vulnerable and tired your body can feel—not to mention the hunger. Many individuals found some great advantages in cardio routines, in fact, several studies have shown that aerobic exercise, such as running, cycling, and high intensity training actually decreases appetite. There are two possible reasons for this. The first one is the release of hormones after exercise that reduce hunger, and the second is post-exercise mood and self-esteem boost, which can improve your motivation to not overeat.

So, how do you combine your new meal plan with a fitness routine to achieve efficient results without stressing your body and your mind?

Here's a step-by-step guide to help you carry on with the intermittent fasting diet without jeopardising your overall wellbeing.

Can you work out while intermittent fasting?

Long story short, Yes. The truth is that your body and your brain work together. It is essential to be in a positive state of mind. Vincent Pedre, M.D., a functional medicine physician who often advises intermittent fasting to his patients, says, "It's necessary to listen to your body."

It just boils down to having a decision that works for you, as it does for most things. The 16:8 plan (where people eat all of their meals in an eight-hour time, then fast for 16 hours) and the 5:2 plan are two separate variations of IF (where people eat 500 to 600 calories for two days per week, then eat normally for the other five). Based on the type of workout you choose and the time of the day you prefer to exercise, you'll need to change your fasting daily plan to get the nutrition your body requires in order to do so.

"If you are too weak to exercise after fasting, take care of your diet and exercise later," Pedre advises. This is especially true when it comes to exercising after a long period without eating. While exercise while fasting has some advantages it also brings some disadvantages.

Benefits of working out while fasted.

If you haven't eaten anything since dinner of the night before, going to your 7 a.m. spin session may be a great idea. This form of cardio done with an empty stomach can potentially help you achieve your weight loss goals.

According to a 2016 study published in the Journal of Nutrition and Metabolism, high intensity cardio executed when fasted, will improve fat oxidation. That means your body is burning fat reserves instead of relying on carbohydrates from your last meal to get the energy it needs. According to a 2017 report published in the Obesity journal, regimented fasting times are more effective than total calorie restriction for weight loss.

Other experiments also shown no distinction in body structure changes between those who exercised out fasted and others who fed before exercise (Journal of the International Society of Sports Nutrition).

Overall, when considering whether or not exercising on an empty stomach is for you, it's important to evaluate how you feel. Don't be afraid to experiment with different daily exercise routines before you find one that works for you and most importantly one that you can stick to.

Things to keep an eye out for.

If you feel strong and reinvigorated while exercising on an empty stomach, that's great, however, if you feel weak or lightheaded, it might be the time for a change in your routine.

"It's true that fasting allows you to lose more weight, but it also allows you to lose more muscle," says Jaime Schehr, N.D., R.D. "When the body's glycogen reserves (aka energy stores) are exhausted, the body will turn to protein for food, which is the very opposite of what most people want."

It's crucial to refurnish your body with carbohydrates and protein (especially after a workout) to help your muscles grow stronger and prevent injury.

So, how do you pick the right workout for your intermittent fasting plan?

When it comes to scheduling your excercises and your intermittent fasting plan, there are few things you may wish to know. There are types of workouts that tends to reduce the muscles faster than others. These routines require a meal consumed right afterward or a higher carbohydrate consumption earlier in the day.

Cardio and HIIT

Fasted cardio, when performed properly, can be an excellent friend to your workout routine. Depending on the kind of exercise you execute, you may or may not need a meal immediately afterward. "I usually advise my clients that if they are performing a high-intensity interval training cardio with a strength-based routine, they shouldn't let pass to much time before they break their fast," Schehr tells mbg. "On the other hand, if it's more of a steady-state aerobic, it doesn't have to be as near to breaking the fast."

If you're out for a slow and steady morning run, you might be able to hold off on eating for a few hours afterward. However, if this makes you feel tired and dizzy, bring with you a meal to consume right after the end your workout. It is important that the combination of your diet and your fitness routine does not affect negatively your health and your ability to carry on with your day.

It's also crucial to ease into every rigorous exercise on this new diet. "If people have a lot of hypoglycemia and don't feel well while they're fasted, it can take some time to ease into fasted cardio," Schehr says. "To be able to reach these fasted conditions, you must train your body correctly." She suggests to gradually increase the intensity of the exercises as the body adjusts itself to working out more quickly.

Strength training

It's very important to fuel the body with protein and complex carbohydrates before and after working out, especially if you want to gain muscle mass. In fact, if you are trying to gain mass and stamina, I would recommend exercising right before you are about to break your fast, otherwise the muscles you worked out during the training won't be able to heal.

When you execute strength exercises during your feeding window, the muscles will have enough fuel to complete the task without breaking down.

It really boils down to what makes you smile the most, says Abby Cannon, J.D., R.D., CDN. "We have to strike a balance; what are the fitness objectives? How do you like to feel during your exercises, and how do you feel during your workout? "she explains. "You know there is something if you find yourself completely exhausted and therefore unable to exercise efficiently. Having a small snack before your workout can help you achieve your weightlifting or HIIT workout goals." In this case, workouts executed in the late afternoon or evening would be a great option for you.

Yoga and low-intensity workouts

Low-intensity exercises, whether fasted or after your meal window, can be a good option for your body during the days you're feeling low on energy or when you're first transitioning to intermittent fasting.

This can be an excellent choice, according to Schehr, if you're looking for a simpler fitness routine to fit into the shortest window of your day.

To get the best out of your fasting plan and your workout routine, you may want to follow this plan or at least, give it a try!

Monday: cardio in the morning, followed by a high-protein meal.

Tuesday: complex carbohydrate brunch, p.m. strength & conditioning, and dinner.

Wednesday: low-intensity exercise (yoga, barre, Pilates, etc.)

Thursday: cardio in the morning, followed by a high-protein meal.

Friday: complex carbohydrate lunch, resistance & conditioning in the afternoon, and dinner

Saturday or Sunday: Yoga, barre, Pilates, or another low-intensity routine.

This plan is based on your own fasting requirements and can be tweaked to suit your needs.

The Super-foods

Intermittent fasting allows you to choose when and what you can eat. Many of the items on this "superfood" list have healthy and important nutrients that help our body to sustain and thrive during a fasting period. An comprehensive study published in the British Medical Journal recently came out, claiming that consuming mostly plant protein lowers your risk of death. Daily consumption of red meat and a heavy intake of animal products has been attributed to many health issues and a reduced life span. On the other hand, a dietary regimen high in plant protein, such as legumes (peas, beans, and lentils), whole grains, and nuts, decreases the possibility of diabetes, heart disease, and stroke. For a longer, healthier, and leaner life, harness the strength of plants!

Phytochemicals (*phyto* comes from the Greek word which stands for for plant), are Mother Nature's medicine cabinet. Phytochemicals is a term used to describe the thousands of nutrients present in edible plants that help our bodies to fight degenerative diseases such as heart disease and cancer. Some foods containing phytochemicals are fruits, berries and whole grains.

Black coffee

I can't stress enough how good black coffee is for your fitness goal and weight loss. Coffee beans are seeds, and like all seeds, they're full of plant compounds. Coffee is, in particular, the single most abundant source of antioxidants in the Western diet. It's what I like to call a "plant juice." Black coffee also contains high levels of: **Vitamin B2**.The same is applicable to decaf coffee as it has the same number of antioxidants as standard coffee. When in doubt choose to buy organic coffee; it's better for your health and for the world we live in. Organic coffee beans are also higher in beneficial antioxidants and chlorogenic acid, which aid in the prevention of type 2 diabetes and the reduction of blood pressure. Many people also detect a change in flavour. Let's not forget that coffe significantly improves your physical performance by increasing Epinephrine (Adrenaline) levels in the blood which translates into a higher level of energy. That is probably why gym trainers suggests to drink a cup before workouts. Not only black coffe increases energy but also improve your mood and your cognitive functioning.

Spinach

Spinach is a nutrient-dense green superfood available in a variety of forms, including raw, frozen, and canned. Spinach, one of the world's healthiest foods, is low in calories but high in nutrients like vitamin C, vitamin A, vitamin K, and essential folate. It's also high in potassium and magnesium, which help to reduce blood pressure.

Quinoa

Quinoa (KEEN-wah) is a superfood packed with vitamins,

minerals, enzymes, and fibre. It's actually different from most grains since it's a whole protein, which means it has the perfect amount of all necessary amino acids the body uses to make new proteins. Quinoa, in particular, has twice the protein of other cereal grains.

Extra-virgin olive oil (EVOO)

Extra-virgin olive oil (EVOO) is high in antioxidants and good fats, studies have shown that it has a variety of health benefits. It is proven to be the only vegetable oil that contains a significant number of disease-fighting polyphenols and anti-inflammatory compounds. Many illnesses, including heart disease, cancer, metabolic syndrome, diabetes, and arthritis, are thought to be caused by chronic inflammation.

Black beans

Beans were once considered subsistence food and poor man's meat, but they are now seen a nutritious staple. Beans are a flexible, hearty, yet ridiculously cheap superfood that Americans have yet to accept. Beans have the highest protein content of any vegetable, and they're also high in minerals, fibre, and essential B vitamins (especially heart-healthy folate). Beans are often high in complex carbohydrates, which have long-lasting nutrition and are considered strong slow carbs.

Dark beans, such as black beans, are among the foods with the highest levels of disease-fighting antioxidants, according to the

United States Department of Agriculture. These little black beauties are high in calcium, plant protein, and fibre, and they also taste delicious! Black beans will satisfy your hunger without emptying your pockets, and they're more common than ever. They should be on everyone's plate at least once a week.

Beets

The humble beet is often underestimated as one of the healthiest plants on the planet, good for the brain and effective at reducing blood pressure. Beets have a great nutritional profile: they're low in calories but high in nutrients like fibre, folate, manganese, potassium, calcium, iron, and vitamin C. Beets are also a good source of nitrates. (Nitrates are converted by the body into nitric oxide, a chemical that aids in blood pressure control and athletic performance.)

Choose the red/purple variety and protect the cells from free radical destruction by eating a normal dose of *anthocyanins* — the blue pigmented polyphenol present in red/purple beets. Beets are fat and cholesterol free, plus they have low salt values. Beets have minimal pesticide residues and are thus safe to purchase also if non-organic.

Nuts and seeds

Superfoods include raw and unsalted walnuts, almonds, and pistachios, as well as chia seeds and ground flaxseeds. For your own wellbeing, essential fatty acids must be included in the diet.

These vital healthy fats, such as omega-3 alpha-linolenic acid, are abundant in both nuts and seeds (ALA). Walnuts and flaxseeds are two ancient plant foods that have nourished humanity since the dawn of civilisation, and they're both high in ALA. Nuts and seeds are also antioxidant powerhouses.

Broccoli

Broccoli is a nutritious powerhouse, packed with vitamins, minerals, fibre, and antioxidants (especially vitamin C). Broccoli is a member of the Brassica oleracea plant family. Cruciferous vegetables include broccoli, Brussels sprouts, kale, and cauliflower, which are all edible plants. This community of vegetables, also known as anti-cancer vegetables, has been shown to successfully treat artery disease and heart vessel damage in diabetics by researchers. Cruciferous vegetables are present in cancer-prevention diets and they can be eaten on a regular basis. Broccoli is a great super-healthy alternative while you are on a fasting regimen because it's low in calories and high in nutrition. Pesticide residue is almost never found on broccoli therefore it is safe to purchase also if non-organic. It's also a food high in prebiotics, or bacteria food, which helps to maintain a balanced gut flora and ncrease the diversity of the beneficial gut bacteria.

Blackberries

Berries are the ultimate anti-aging superfood overall. Blackberries, in particular, contain a variety of essential nutrients such as potassium, magnesium, and calcium, as well as vitamins A, C, E, calcium, iron, and the majority of B vitamins. They're also high in anthocyanins, the pigments that gives blackberries their deep purple hue.

One cup of raw blackberries contains 60 calories, 30 milligrammes of vitamin C, and 8 grammes of dietary fibre in a megadose (one serving of blackberries delivers 31 percent of your daily dietary fibre needs). Blackberries, whether fresh or frozen, are a real superfood that should be on your weekly menu. If organic is available, I highly recommend buying it.

Lentils

This powerful legume is rich in fibre and protein, and it enhances the flavour and texture of every dish. Lentils are sometimes used as a meat substitute in conventional dishes by vegans and vegetarians; however, unlike animal protein, lentils are fat and cholesterol free. Lentils have a protein content of more than 25%. They're also a good source of iron, which is also deficient in vegetarian diets. Lentils are low in calories, high in iron and folate, and an ideal source of additional nutrients. They are both cheap and easy to prepare, they should be the first thing on your shopping list!

Lentils don't need to be soaked and they cook quickly, anywhere from 10 to 25 minutes depending on the variety. You can also buy precooked lentils, which are delicious and help you to save time in the kitchen.

CHAPTER FOUR

Intermittent Fasting May Affect Men And Women Differently

Intermittent fasting might not be as effective for some women as it is for men, according to some evidence. In a study, women's blood sugar control deteriorated after three weeks of intermittent fasting, while men's blood sugar control increased.

There have also been several anecdotal accounts about women's menstrual cycles shifting since they started intermittent fasting. Since female bodies are particularly susceptible to calorie restriction, such changes tend to arise.

If you lower your calories intake too much, it can affect a small portion of the brain called the hypothalamus. This will interact with gonadotropin-releasing hormone (GnRH) secretion, a hormone that helps release two reproductive hormones: luteinizing hormone (LH) and follicle-stimulating hormone (FSH) (FSH). You run the risk of irregular cycles, miscarriage, low bone health and other health consequences as these hormones do not interact with the ovaries.While no similar human trials have been performed, rat experiments have shown that 3-6 months of alternate-day fasting in female rats caused a decline in ovary size and erratic reproductive cycles. A modified solution to intermittent fasting, such as shorter fasting times and fewer days of fasting, should be considered by women for these reasons.

Menopause and Intermittent Fasting

When a woman enters her 40s and 50s during menopause, sex hormones gradually decrease and the ovaries tend to stop processing oestrogen and progesterone, this prevents menstruation. Is is said of a woman to have entered menopause when she has not had a cycle for 12 straight months, but amenorrhea is far from being the only sign of menopause.

Menopause includes a number of effects, including hot spells, vaginal dryness, nausea, diminished libido, brain fog, exhaustion, chills, night sweats, changes in mood, and an elevated risk of heart disease, which can vary from person to person. For some women, there is often a marked difference in metabolism, which usually slows down when oestrogen and progesterone levels get out of control, causing weight gain.

Women can often become less receptive to insulin after menopause as if the other signs were not enough, and they may have trouble absorbing sugar and processed carbohydrates; this physiological transition is called insulin resistance, which also comes with fatigue and sleep problems.

Menopause is a strange and terrifying time in the life of many women. They will no longer feel confident in their bodies and may have problems in identifying with them. Symptoms such as sudden weight gain and brain fog may cause feelings of fear, confusion, anger, tension, and depression.

Fortunately, women can use intermittent fasting as a method to help them handle the sloping roller coaster of menopause. You may want to consider giving it a try if you are dealing with exhaustion, weight gain or insulin resistance during your menopause journey.

Fasting enhances insulin sensitivity, and makes the body absorb sugar and carbohydrates more effectively, reducing the risk of heart disease, diabetes, and other metabolic diseases. It has proven to increase self-esteem, minimise depression and stress, and encourage more positive psychological improvements. Fasting has been shown to help shield brain cells from stress, clean out waste products, restore, and increase their performance.

So yes, menopause might be a tough time for most women, but by eating the right food and adopt some behavioural adjustments, you can control better the symptoms. You can remain fit, comfortable, and healthy even when the hormones are messing with you!

What Causes Menopause Weight Gain?

Weight gain is particularly normal in women over 40, but there is still a controversy about the precise cause and the effects. Lower levels of oestrogen can mean a lower metabolic rate, which, even though our diet has not changed, may lead to weight gain. Basically, since your body change a new dietary regimen has to be adopted in order to sustain your new metabolism. Because of enhanced insulin tolerance, we could be less able to use starches and sugars. Or it may be the two fat-storing and fat-synthesis enzymes, which are more active in postmenopausal women, causing menopause weight gain. Or it's muscle mass reduction that allows them to burn less calories, even at rest. Many women are frustratingly struggling with a rise in ghrelin, the hormone of starvation, and/or a decline in leptin, the hormone that warns us when we are sated.

Remind yourself that weight gain is a common aspect in women's life and might occur for many different and complex reasons. Your weight doesn't say anything about your value and should not be perceived as a failure. It is important you don't lose your willpower during the journey as hormones have much more control on our mindset and on our body mechanisms than we can imagine. Keep in mind that low estrogen levels will make weight management far more difficult. Just don't beat yourself up because not only it doesn't burn calories but it is also self-defeating.

How can intermittent fasting help with menopause weight gain?

The total amount of calories you eat has to be limited. In order to result in weight loss, having a calorie deficit is in fact crucial. This can be even more helpful during menopause since due to hormonal fluctuations, ageing, poor sleep, excessive weight gain is a common enemy for women.

A 2017 research states that women's energy consumption after menopause decreases by about 650 calories therefore your diet needs to be adapted. Intermittent fasting can also slow down the process of ageing of tissues and has proven itself as a fairly simple approach to improving the quality of life for women during the postmenopausal period.

Bottom line: After menopause, shall you consider intermittent fasting?

This dietary regimen is considered by many a wonderful method for controlling weight gain, insulin resistance, and other typical menopausal symptoms. Having said that, some people are still reluctant when it comes to fasting. This restrictive meal plan might put your body under moderate discomfort and preassure, so if you suffer from adrenal exhaustion or any chronic condition, you should consider your options before starting.

If you finally decide to give intermittent fasting a shot, it is essential you pay attention to how you feel and how your body reacts day by day. You may want to either shorten your fasting or miss a fasting slot if the regimen is too restrictive for you.

Remember, you can always start slow and see how you handle it!

PRACTICAL REMINDERS FOR EVERY WOMAN GOING THROUGH MENOPAUSE

Keep Yourself Cool

Sweaty nights and hot flashes are no jokes. It's best to have a tool on hand to stay calm as they hit you in the middle of the night. And, of course, by "tool," we mean a bed fan with a wireless remote. It is precisely engineered to spread the much-needed cool air directly between your sheets.

Meditate And Breathe Away Pain

Menopause symptoms can get worse because of stress. According to the Mayo Clinic, relaxing is key. They recommend finding a peaceful spot and try diaphragmatic breathing for 5 to 10 minutes. This technique involves fully engaging the abdominal muscles, the stomach and the diaphragm when breathing. Most of the movement happens in the belly area rather than in the chest.

Now place your right hand on your stomach and your left hand on your chest. Tray to breath as you would normally do, you may notice your chest does all the work while in diaphragmatic breathing it's different. When you inhale your belly rises and your left hand will come up, when you exhale, tighten your stomach muscles and let the belly sinks down together with your hand. The hand on top of the belly will help you understand if the practice is done correctly as you will have a visual proof (your hand going up and down) that you are doing it correctly.

Try to make this practice ad habit, it is proven to have many benefit since the air you breath goes straight into your belly.

First, as we just said, this practice helps you relax by lowering the levels of cortisol (the stress hormone) in your body. Second, it slows down your heart rate and because of that it lowers your blood pressure. It is shown to improve core muscle stability and to withstand more exercise. This breathing is in fact commonly performed during yoga and pilates classes. Lastly, diaphragmatic breathing really does minimise pain.

Go Natural

Many women have considered essential oils to be effective in relieving the effects of menopause. Keep a roller bottle filled with diluted peppermint oil next to your bed for relief from night sweats. I also suggest keeping one in your everyday bag for on-the-go relief. A diffuser is also a calming option to keep the space quiet and relaxed, but remember not to use it for more than 20 to 30 minutes every 2 hours.

Change Up Your Diet And Try Intermittent Fasting

For postmenopausal women, intermittent fasting may be particularly effective for weight management and weight loss. There are various ways of intermittent fasting, many of which include reducing the calorie consumption for a certain amount of time.

Embrace Exercise

After menopause, women's bodies will change radically. A recent study showed that menopause can change the way oxygen is used by women's muscles. These muscles' shifts translates into a higher necessity of exercising. Working out can also help with some of the most common symptoms, such as mood swings, and exhaustion.

Don't be afraid to Experiment

Vaginal wall thinness and a reduction in normal lubrication can be caused by hormone changes and physical changes during menopause. This can also result in a natural decline in libido. It's important to respect what works for your relationship, but sexual toys might be the solution if you and your partner want to get things going in the bedroom again. Studies have shown that, with the advent of vibrators, many women had great results in increasing their libido and sexual pleasure. One precious thing I've learned myself: there's no shame in making your partner aware of this aspect of your life and the situation you are going through. There are several types of toys available, talk to your partner and try those that suits you better!

Use The Power Of Your Mind

There is a multitude of websites that offer medical informations, studies, and products that convince women menopause is not something you should be scared of. It is a natural aspect of the life cycle and as such, try to consider it as a new phase of your life, not something you need to stop or undo. Nothing is wrong with menopause, or with you. As you step through the transition, accepting this new situation will also help frame your experience.

Health Benefits of Intermittent Fasting for Women

Yes, intermittent fasting is a great way to finally achieve your body goals and control your weight but there's so much more. This dietary regimen is a great friend for your health since it significantly lowers the risk of contracting chronic diseases.

• Cardiovascular Wellbeing

The main cause of death worldwide is heart failure and high blood pressure, high LDL cholesterol, high triglyceride levels are three of the most important risk factors for cardiac failure.

in a sample of 16 obese men and women it has been shown that intermittent fasting decreases blood pressure by 6% in just eight weeks. It also cuts LDL cholesterol and triglycerides by 25%, according to the same report. However, the data concerning the correlation between intermittent fasting and improved levels of LDL cholesterol and triglycerides is not quite consistent.

A review of 40 normal-weight individuals showed that four weeks of intermittent fasting did not result in a decrease in LDL cholesterol or triglycerides. Until researchers can completely comprehend the impact of intermittent fasting on cardiac health, higher-quality studies with more rigorous methods are needed.

• Diabetes risks

Intermittent fasting will also help to effectively control and reduce the risk of developing diabetes. The diet tends to decrease some of the risk factors for diabetes, comparable to constant calorie restriction. It does so primarily by reducing the amount of insulin and reducing the response to insulin.

Six months of intermittent fasting decreased insulin levels by 29% and insulin tolerance by 19% in a randomised controlled trial of more than 100 overweight or obese women. The levels of blood sugar remained the same.

What's more, in patients with pre-diabetes (a disease in which blood sugar levels are elevated but not high enough to diagnose diabetes) 8-12 weeks of intermittent fasting resulted in reducing insulin levels by 20-31 percent and blood sugar levels by 3-6 percent.

However, in terms of blood sugar, intermittent fasting can not be as effective for women as it is for men.

A small study showed that after 22 days of alternate-day fasting, blood sugar management for women worsened, although there was no adverse effect on male blood sugar. Despite this side effect, the decrease in insulin and insulin tolerance will likely reduce the risk of diabetes, particularly in pre-diabetic individuals.

• **Weight Loss**

When done right, intermittent fasting can be an quick and efficient way to lose weight, since short-term fasts can help you eat less calories. A variety of studies show that intermittent fasting is as effective for short-term weight loss as conventional calorie-restricted diets. A 2018 study of overweight adult trials showed that intermittent fasting resulted in an average weight loss of 15 lbs (6.8 kg) over the course of 3-12 months.

In overweight or obese adults for a span of 3-24 weeks, another review found that intermittent fasting decreased body weight by 3-8 percent. Participants lowered their waist circumference by 3-7 percent during the same time span. It's worth noting that the long-term consequences of intermittent fasting on female weight loss are also unclear.

Intermittent starvation tends to assist with weight loss in the short term. The amount you lose, though, will possibly depend on the number of calories you eat during times of non-fasting and how long you stick to the lifestyle.

• **Decreasing Appetite**

Switching to intermittent fasting may help you eat less naturally. One research showed that while participants' food consumption was reduced to a four-hour duration, young men ate 650 fewer calories per day. A further research looked at the impact of a long, 36-hour fast on eating habits of 24 healthy men and women. While eating more calories on the post-fast day, their overall calorie balance fell by 1,900 calories. A substantial decrease.

OTHER HEALTH BENEFITS

A variety of human and animal studies indicate that other health benefits can also be obtained from intermittent fasting.

- **Inflammation reduction**: Prolonged fasting has been proved minimise essential indicators of inflammation. Chronic inflammation can contribute to weight gain and numerous health issues.

- **Increased psychological Well-being**: One research showed that stress and binge eating habits were diminished by eight weeks of intermittent fasting while enhancing body appearance in obese adults.

- **Increased longevity**: Intermittent fasting increases lifespan by 33-83% in rats and mice. The effect on human survival has yet to be calculated.

- **Preserve muscle mass**: In contrast to constant calorie restriction, intermittent fasting tends to be more efficient at maintaining muscle mass. Having a greater muscle mass means that your body needs more energy to function and this will increase your daily calories intake. The difference between fat and lean mass is a question of tissue maintenance. Muscles are dynamic tissues which are constantly working and require more energy in order to sustain themselves. Fat, on the other hand, is a passive reserve of energy which we don't normally use and that does not require a significant calories consumption.

- **Cancer Protection**: Several studies have shown that by reducing lymphoma growth, limiting tumour survival, and slowing the spread of cancer cells, alternate-day fasting can decrease cancer danger.

- **Lower chance of inflammation**: Obesity can lead to skin conditions that are uncomfortable.

- **Lower depression rates**: Obesity often lead to loneliness, a decreased sense of the self, and depression. Taking control of your weight and accepting your body will highly influence your life.

The benefits of intermittent fasting for women may extend beyond the colories restriction. Although some medical experts argue that this dietary plan succeeds only because it allows individuals to reduce food consumption and so, calories intake, others disagree. They states that with the same number of calories and nutrients, intermittent fasting leads to greater results than mere conventional restrictive meal schedules.

HEALTHY DIET TIPS FOR WOMEN AFTER 50

I can imagine all of this can be new for you and it might seems challenging if you never approached diets or fitness routines. What's important is that you are motivated to succede. You can start slow, some people needs some time in order to get used to an healthier lifestyle and say goodbye to bad habits.

1. Start by Walking: There is conflict about whether walking is as good as running for you, but everyone acknowledges that it is incredibly good for your health to exercise consistently even at a slow speed. Walking at a brisk pace for one to 2.5 hours per week cuts the chance of death by 25%.

2. Workout on a Daily Basis: Once you start to feel healthier and leaner, regular exercise will be incredibly helpful to maintain your progress. There are classes for senior people online that works just fine, but you can also find several gyms with live classes in your area. For older adults who never exercised it is particularly important to be followed by a competent instructur. You may want to consider having a personal trainer for the first few months. This will motivate you even further.

3. Eat the Right Foods: Building muscle is a vital aspect of reducing weight. However, you'll require stamina. Lean mass in fact demands a good amount of digested and synthetized proteins in order to grow. By reducing unhealthy foods and increasing

protein it's easy to eat nutritious and living a healthy lifestyle. This includes regularly consuming fruits, vegetables, whole grains, and unprocessed lean meats in your daily meal plan. Most of these foods are high in fiber, vitamins and contains numerous antioxidants. Never forget to consume nuts and seeds, even if they are high in calories they help you lose weight. They are rich of magnesium and vitamin E. Since they requires zero preparation they are a delicious and filling alternative for your snacks. I also love to add them to my salads.

5. Portion Control: As a general rule, every decade of your life, you need about 100 fewer calories a day. If you didn't know it, you are potentially eating in a way that wasn't in line with your actual biological reality. By reducing portion sizes, you can manage food consumption without having to over exercise.

Most of the time, life is an option, a choice we make everyday based on our actions. Deciding to eat better is deciding to live better... and longer! Embracing the opportunities of ageing rather than focus on the limits is the secret to losing weight after 50.

I like to call this process *life-gaining* rather than *weight-losing*. Intermittent fasting is not a magic weight-loss formula, it takes effort and motivation, a good amount of strength and resilience to achieve your goals.

Dipping a Toe in the Water

It's easy to go for at least 12 hours without eating. Just sleep, maybe dream about having the dinner you skipped. But when you wake you are done, or very close to 12 hours. Or you can just having your regular dinner, go to sleep and skip breakfast, extending the fast until lunch.

If, after having missed dinner, you spend a good night time, if when you wake up you're not hungry, postpone breakfast slightly longer, until you can reach a 14 hour fasting.

Try to feed in between meals as little as possible. Ignore short, frequent meals throughout the day, if your body is not screaming for it. Eat meals with enough calories that can make you go through the same hours relatively effortlessly for lunch and dinner, avoiding snacking in between.

If you can't not introduce something in your stomach, it is perfectly understandable. Here, juices might come to your help. If you're trying a strict liquid diet, increase the number of liquid-based meals to two per day. It may be a delicious soup or a refreshing smoothie! (Don't forget to add your proteins).

Minimize calories intake directly after exercise and restrict whey protein, which is repeatedly seen as an optimizer of muscle protein synthesis. Carbohydrate consumption may reduce GH output.

If you've overindulged the night before, working out at a high intensity whilst fasted will help you shed overweight.

This applies if you workout less than an hour a day. If you are extremely active and need to recover repeatedly from one series of exercise in order to prepare for a second during the day, or the day after, you might need more carbohydrates to not deplete your stocks.

Before starting, I assume deep down you all have a question. Is prolonged fasting a good way to eat for a woman who passed her 50th year of age? Bear in mind that you're just expected to fast for 12 to 16 hours, not for many consecutive days. You still have plenty of time to enjoy a balanced and rewarding diet.

Of course, if you're confronting precarious metabolic conditions or prescription guidelines, you may need to eat daily on your schedule, and the fasting needs to be checked very closely. You can speak to your doctor about the healthier dietary habits for you, before making any adjustments to your life.

CHAPTER FIVE

Nutritional Rules For Intermittent Fasting

When I first started learning about intermittent fasting, several years ago, every piece of information that I could find online or in books was about the fasting phase rather than the actual meal plan and what is recommended to eat during this dietary regimen.

When you are restricting your daily calories intake, what you eat is much more important! Make sure you are not depriving your organism from vital vitamins, nutrients, fats, and proteins that it requires to sustain a healthy immune system, recover from injury or disease, keep muscles solid, and keep the metabolism working smoothly. I believe what we eat can deeply influence our life and our health. I decided to include some diet secrets that I have been following since day one as well as realistic fasting schedules and recipes to assist you.

RULE 1: ONLY EAT REAL FOOD

This means no counterfeit food and no diet-drinks. Chances are you have fond memories of neon orange corn chips, fizzy drinks and sugar packed candies. Hopefully, things have changed and you're enjoying big bowls of rocket and Parmesan salads, roasted artichoke and monkfish. However, the majority of people, follow a diet that is rich in refined, low-fiber, and nutrient-deficient foods.

Keep in mind that not all processed food is evil. Food without added sugar or salt and freshly-frozen fruit and vegetables are still a good alternative.

Pay attention to labels that shouts "fat 0%" because that fat is simply substituted with refined sugars (apart from dairy products, where low fat is fine). Most sources of sugar, such as sucrose, maltose, glucose, fructose are all bad for your diet and for your health.

Highly processed foods may also have high levels of chemicals which can have a blocking effect on hormones that regulate weight loss. My advice? When in doubt, keep the meals genuine!

What Makes Up a Real-Food Diet?

• **Protein**

Amino acids, also known as the "*building blocks of life*", are what makes up proteins. They are also vital for the synthesis of hormones and neurotransmitters. We know there are approximately 500 amino acids present in nature, only 20 of them are crucial for our body. These can be divided into essential amino acids (9) and non essential amino acids (11). Animal protein such as meat, dairy, fish, and egg contain all the amino acids required.

Yes, before you start bulling eggs, just know they are a great option that has to be present in your diet. One egg yolk has 200 mg of cholesterol which makes them the greater source of cholesterol in our diet but remember, there is only a tiny correlation between dietary cholesterol and blood cholesterol. It has been scientifically proven that one egg per day does not influence your heart health.

Also, eggs are low in saturated fat which means you are less likely to feel hunger later in the day if you eat eggs for breakfast. On the other hand, incomplete proteins have vegetable origins (except for soybeans, they are the only vegetable protein with the same characteristics of animal proteins). You can get your protein from almonds, peas, legumes and grains if you are vegetarian or vegan, but you need a wide selection of these foods to ensure you get the full spectrum of necessary amino acids into your body.

Top tip, increase the amount of beans and lentils in your diet. Kidney beans, butter beans, chickpeas or red and green lentils are a fantastic alternative to meat. They're high in protein and contain complex carbohydrates, which release energy slowly and gradually during the day. They also provide fibres that may help to balance the fats in your blood. Consume them as you like, you can make stews, casseroles, soups, and salads.

Every Meal Should Contain Protein

You may have seen people eating a banana or enjoying a smoothie while waiting for dinner. There is nothing wrong with this, but in order to balance your blood sugar it is better to consume some protein, preferably around 1/2 oz to 1 oz (10-30 g). You can make a sandwich with a few extra slices of ham or add protein powder into your smoothie. These are full protein sources to have on hand that can be stored in the fridge and easily used to make a complete nutritious snack. Boiled eggs, roast beef, cooked/tinned soybeans, chicken, canned fish (like tuna, mackerel, or sardines), cottage cheese, quark and salmon are also decent sources of proteins that you may want to consider.

What Is a Good Source of Protein?

When it comes to the influence of several protein sources on our metabolism and on energy consumption, researches are showing a difference between them. Nutrition from animal products, such as beef, eggs, milk, poultry, seafood, and shellfish, provides all of the essential amino acids, which the body cannot produce on its own. Animal proteins, rich in fat provide more energy than proteins produced from vegetarian sources. Beans, nuts, berries, lentils, peas, lettuce, vegetables, rice, and other vegetarian protein sources are rich in fibre and anti-nutrients, which delay protein breakdown. In essence, only 80-90 percent of vegetarian forms of protein are broken down, which means that you need to consume plenty to achieve the same effect on the body as animal proteins. You can still will lose weight, but it will be due to muscle loss rather than fat loss.

Whey and casein are milk proteins that tend to have an especially beneficial impact on weight. Soy protein (found in soy milk, tofu, and protein powder, for example) is another type of protein that aids with weight loss in addition to its protein content. The soybean is not only the legume with the most protein, but it also has the best protein content in the vegetarian realm. During dieting and calorie restriction, soy will sustain the development of thyroid hormone. When you eat less calories, your thyroid hormone levels decrease, allowing your metabolism to slow down, but consumption of soy can counter this.

• **Carbohydrates**

In diet and weight loss, carbs are one of the most contentious subjects. We have been advised for years that we can eat so much fat and that the primary source of heart disease is saturated fat. However, some scientists have recently disputed this assumption, arguing that carbs are especially to blame for the obesity crisis and a slew of other diseases.

The body searches for calories in its glycogen reserves while it is starved of carbohydrates. Fats (the good ones) and healthy carbs are needed. It's useless and potentially risky to completely avoid carbohydrates. Not all carbohydrates are in fact equal. Carbohydrates with a low caemic index (GI) found in fiber-rich fruits, beans, unrefined grains and vegetables are important to maintain an healthy organism and can, for example, actively promote weight loss by decreasing appetite. On the other hand, High-GI processed carbs, such as those found in soft drinks, white bread, pastries, some breakfast cereals and sweeteners, has to be avoided since they can affect long-term health. Studies proved that the risk of heart failure and type 2 diabetes rises when eating a lot of high-GI carbohydrates.

In recent years, there has been a lot of studies on low-carbohydrate diets. Initially, it was believed they could affect bone and kidney health, but this theory has been denied quite quickly. Low-carb diets can be beneficial for weight loss and can reduce the risk factors for heart disease and diabetes. They do, though, come with threats too.

First of all, a low intake of carbs (those deriving from fruits, vegetables and whole grains) translates into an insufficiency of certain vitamins and minerals, particularly folates, which are essential for women who wants to get pregnant. Second, by leaving out unrefined sugars, this regimen significantly decreases the amount of fibre, which can led to constipation. This can raise the risk of colorectal cancer in the long run. Finally, a low-carb, animal-protein-based diet has been linked to a slightly higher risk of mortality. High consumption of meat and dietary products contain compounds that are inflammatory, called prostaglandins. For the body, inflammation is bad news. The most common side effects of an extremely low-carb diet are poor breath, mood swings, constipation and nausea. There are definitely healthier ways to lose weight without compromising your organism.

Today, the abundance of slow-acting carbohydrates permeates a great variety of food; with just a bit of dietary knowledge, it is easy to eat correctly. Some examples of healthy sources of carbohydrates are unsweetened whole-grain bread (preferably sourdough), slow-cooked whole wheat pasta, slow-cooked brown rice, whole-grain flakes (such as oat porridge), unsweetened muesli, all sorts of fruits and vegetables (including bananas!), berries, mushrooms, legumes (beans, peas, lentils), grains, seeds, and root vegetables (even boiled potatoes).

Long story short, choose protein over carbs as they prolong the feeling of fullness as they slow down the absorption of carbohydrates and fats. This will lead to a steady blood-sugar curve and a lower insulin production. You should still eat all of the three (protein, carbs and fats) in the right measure. Balance, after all, is always the key to success. Mix these main nutrients in your recipes, but don't forget: Carbs are also present in fruit and vegetables, so you do not need to eat a pile of noodles or potatoes!

Carbohydrate that prevent fat burning are basically foods that have a high GI content, where quantity plays an important part. A little candy won't have any effect on your weight loss journey, but a big bag of sugar packed snacks will ruin all your efforts. Soda, squash, desserts, ice cream, biscuits, sweets, white bread, cornflakes, french fries, cheese doodles, and many types of crispy bread (a healthy crispy bread would have seeds and/or whole grains in/on it) are all foods with a high GI and a lot of carbohydrates.

• **Fat**

Since fat is the most caloric nutrient, regulating and controlling your fat consumption will help you in your battle for weight loss. Fat, however, plays a crucial part in every diet because it contains the essential acids required for the absorption of vitamins. A lack of fats in one's diet can contribute to a number of health issues. If you consume the right kinds of fat in the right quantities, fats will make you feel full longer. That's why I son't want you to think of fat as your enemy, but more as a supporting friend in your search for a healthy lifestyle! Adding a little of the right fat to your meals assists in nutrient absorption and, some would say, increases the taste of your food. Monounsaturated fats or oils (such as olive oil and rapeseed oil) are safer for your heart. As it is heat-stable, coconut oil can be a decent option for cooking too.

Increase the consumption of essential fats by consuming at least two servings of oily fish per week. Mackerel, sardines, tuna, and pilchards are some examples. Omega 3 is a form of polyunsaturated fat contained in oily fish that helps protect against heart disease. Use flaxseed oil in the salad dressing and snack on walnuts if you do not eat seafood.

Some tips:

1. As a low-fat alternative to unhealthy foods, consider lean meat and seafood.

2. Select dairy foods with lower sugar, such as skimmed or semi-skimmed milk and natural yoghurt with reduced fat.

3. Instead of frying or boiling with oil or other fats, roast, poach, or microwave bake.

4. Be careful of smooth sauces and salad dressings. Substitute

with tomato-based sauces. To improve flavour, apply basil, lemon, cloves and garlic to reduced-fat meals. Soy sauce is a great alternative, just remember to choose unsalted soy sauce to avoid adding extra salt to your meal. Remember that even if salt is an important nutrient for our organism and we shouldn't cut it completely from our meals, it's important that we limit our intake. Too much salt can contribute to high blood pressure as it holds excess fluid in the body.

5. Using cheese as a garnish rather than a main course; in other words, no macaroni and cheese! Choose a strong-flavored cheese, such as Parmesan or goat's cheese, so that you only need a limited amount.

• **Coconut**

Coconut oil is very healthy for your wellbeing and for managing your weight. Coconut oil is great whether you're trying to bake, wok, or deep fry something, and can be purchased in your local supermarket. It's a processed fat, of course, which means you remove any antioxidants, but given the large amount of saturated fats in coconut, since it's refined, there are virtually no trans fats. When rapeseed oil is distilled and made odourless and colourless, for example, 12 to 2 percent of trans fats are produced, which isn't ideal. If you want the most natural fat, in health food markets, you can look for cold-pressed coconut fat, but it's fairly pricey and tastes like coconut, which may not be for anyone's tastes. For frying, I use refined coconut oil, and it's the obvious option if you're making popcorn at home.

Eat raw, shredded, or grated coconut. It is tasty and coconut is also perfect for snacking or as part of your meal. Few raw foods taste this delicious, in my opinion! Grated coconut is suitable to bake, to add to fruit salads, and, to be mixed with muesli. Coconut milk is also a perfect addition to a number of dishes, including stews, soups, sauces, and baked goods.

• **Fruit**

Some people say that fruits can make you gain weight. They guarantee that weight gain can be caused even by a modest intake. Most people with a clear understanding of nutrition, however, are conscious that this is not entirely true. As always, balance is key. Carbohydrates (10-20%), water, fibres, vitamins, enzymes, minerals, and other nutrients are all contained in berries. Carbs are the only thing that adds to nutrition, and since most fruits produce only around 10 percent, to get 31⁄2 oz (100 g) of carbs, you will need to consume 2.2 lb (1 kg) of apples. You will only need about 7 oz (a few hundred grammes) and about 10 oz (300 g) of pasta to get the same amount of carbs through bread (cooked). Since more than that is used by the brain only (an average of 4 1⁄2 oz [120-130 g] of carbohydrates every day), eating a significant quantity of fruit per day is not an issue.

Of course, you can only eat so much of something, even fruit, but we're talking about multiple pounds a day here. Personally, every day I try to eat around 1 pound (1⁄2 kg) of fruit, but I'm not afraid to eat twice that amount either. Modern study indicates that the more overweight individuals eat fruit, the more they lose weight. Also people of medium weight will benefit from fruit eating as it helps to defend against adding unnecessary weight. 100% fruit juice, according to one study, also does not induce weight gain. This is most likely due to the high levels of antioxidants, vitamins, and minerals, as well as the fibres that assist in weight reduction.

What Is So Frightening About Fruit?

Those who have a bad opinion about fruits are actually scared about sugar or fructose contained in fruits. A very high intake of fructose is of course an occurrence to avoid, because this is still sugar that needs to be converted into the liver, but I believe you can safely bite into a juicy apple without worrying too much about it. Around half of the fruit sugar is made up of fructose, meaning you get about 50 g (1.75 oz) of fructose for a few pounds of fruit a day. The liver will take up to 75 g (21⁄2 oz) of carbohydrates, and since you rarely consume more than a few pounds of fruit at a time, fructose from is hardly ever an issue.

Artificially inserted fructose, on the other hand, is a different matter. If you use fructose as a sweetener, eat fructose-sweetened sweets, or drink soda with a lot of fructose-rich corn syrup (which is particularly popular in the United States), you can quickly eat more than the liver can tolerate. If this is the case the wastes are turned into fat.

Olive Oil vs. Sunflower Oil and Linseed Oil

Olive oil is well known for its role in the Mediterranean diet, renowned for its heart-healthy qualities, and the property of decreasing risks of type 2 diabetes and of some forms of cancer. New research has shown that the benefits of olive oil also extend into the metabolic realm. It alsocontains antioxidants, and extremely high levels of monounsaturated fats (in the form of 70-80% oleic acid). Oleuropein (a polyphenol) is one of these, and it has been shown in rats to boost the ability to turn body fat to gas. This suggests that even though they did not exercise more than the other rats, rats that were given olive oil were in better condition than those that were not fed any. It's uncertain what happens to a person's metabolism when they eat oleuropein, but it seems that the fat in olive oil is one of the simplest to burn. During exercise oleic acid leaves the fat cells more quickly and gets metabolised.

In one study, among groups who consumed olive oil, sunflower oil, or linseed oil, researchers compared metabolism after the administration. The oil that improved metabolism the most was olive oil, followed by sunflower oil, and eventually linseed oil. Oleic acid in olive oil (monounsaturated omega-9 fat), linoleic acid in sunflower oil (polyunsaturated omega-6 fat) and alfalinolenic acid in linseed oil are the principal fatty acids in these three aliments (polyunsaturated omega-3 fat).

Olive Oil vs. Cream

An Australian research looked at the impact on fat burning of calories from fat after breakfast, with the main fat coming from olive oil or cream. Fat burning was assessed five hours after the meal and for those who were given olive oil, it was found to be slightly higher. Also a higher appetite was found in those individuals, but only for those with the heaviest body weight. Looking at these conclusion it's worth noting that dairy products, such as cream, are not the worst aliment for your body weight. Dairy fats include around 25 percent SCT and MCT, the most readily burnt types of saturated fats. Besides, there is a fair number of monounsaturated fats as well as CLA (Conjugated Linoleic Acid) in milk fats. Olive oil fat is still to be preferred to any fat coming form beef or pork.

• Whole Grain

We may count whole grain bread, whole wheat noodles, whole grain cereals and brown rice among the variety of whole grain products, as well as flax seeds, quinoa, oatmeal, barley and rye. For all these products, the common denominator is that the seed/grain preserves the bran (the "shell") and includes fibre, vitamin B, and trace elements. Moreover, the part known as germ, is rich in vitamins and antioxidants. Refined foods preserve only the endosperm, which includes only starch, protein, and a slight amount of fat, as well as fragments of fibre, vitamins, minerals, and antioxidants. Whole grain alternatives should be favoured over processed grain alternatives for genuinely healthy food. There's one downside to big quantities of whole grain, though: sensitive stomachs can suffer, so a balance has to be found to not overdo your whole grain intake. Consuming whole grains is healthy both for your wellbeing and for your weight. They are digested more slowly than refined one, keeping the levels of insulin and sugar down.

Weight Loss Promoted by Whole Grain

Because all grain options contain 5-8 percent less calories on average than their processed counterparts, a portion of the same size would yield less fat. Although 5% less calories does not sound like much, if you eat 2,500 kcal a day and 40% of those calories come from carbohydrates such as grains and seeds, you would be saving about 50 kcal per day (as long as you manage to consume as many of the whole grain varieties as you can). By eating 50 kcal less per day, 90% of those who tend to gain weight can get rid of it in relatively little time. A study has shown that women whose diets includes whole grainsrare half as likely to gain weight over a 12-year period as those who eat the least whole grains.

Whole grain improves metabolism

Whole grain and food with high-quality ingredients raise your metabolism more than processed food. The rise in metabolism after a snack consisting of either white bread with refined cheese (such as margarine cheese or cream cheese) or whole-grain bread with standard cheese was compared in an exciting report. Likewise the weight, protein and carbohydrates, the caloric consumption remained the same. After this, researchers measured the metabolism of the subject over six hours and concluded that a significantly higher metabolism was caused by the whole grain bread and the cheese. In fact, whole grain bread increased metabolism by twice as much as white bread. A total of 19.9 percent of the energy content of all grain breads went to food digestion, while white bread only required 10.7 percent of the energy content of the meals. This means that you will see a change in your waistline if you eat whole grain bread instead of white bread every day.

RULE 2: SKIP THE SUGAR

Sugar makes you obese and encourages your skin to age prematurely. Sugar is associated with collagen and elastin and decreases skin elasticity, making you look older than your age. To add a little flavour, the recipes I include in this book use low-sugar fruits and the occasional drizzle of a natural sweetener such as honey, which is perfect and tastes amazing. Sugar is usually harmful for you and you must quit it.

If you need a sweet fix, stick to dark chocolate. You will need less that your normal super processed sweet to feel satisfied and happy.

RULE 3: WATCH THE ALCOHOL

The alcohol level in most alcoholic beverages has risen over time. Remember that a drink will have more alcohol than you may think. Two units may be contained in a tiny glass of wine (175ml/5 1/2fl oz/ cup). Alcohol, beside not being the best companion of life, brings with it useless calories, so if you're looking to lose weight, consider cutting it down, or better yet, don't drink any. For a woman the a limit is two units of alcohol per day; for a male, three units can suffice. A single pub measure (25ml/3/4fl oz) of alcohol, for example, is around one unit, and one or one and a half units is half a pint of lager, wine, bitter or beer.

So if you can't miss the thrill of holding the glass in your hand, you'd better enjoy a soft drink or an alcohol-free grape juice as a delightful wine alternative. Alcohol-free drinks are becoming more and more popular.

RULE 4: EAT FRUIT, DON'T DRINK IT

If you drink 1 litre (35fl oz/4 cups) of fruit juice, bear in mind that you'll be eating 500 calories. That's good if you're fasting with juice, but too much if it's just a snack. For the same number of calories, you might eat a baked potato with tuna and two slices of fruit.

Pick herbal teas (especially green tea, which may aid fat loss) instead. You are welcome to have a cup of tea or coffee. Usually in most intermittent fasting plan there are tiny quantities of milk allowed, but hold it to a splash.

When fasting drink lots of water, try to go for a fluid consumption of 1.22 litres (4070fl oz/ 8 cups) each day. Not only can this serve to keep hunger pangs at bay, but it will keep you hydrated as well.

RULE 5: AVOID THE PITFALLS

1. When you begin fasting, you may feel hungry at those times when you would usually feed, especially if you used to eat sugary snacks. You may feel light-headed, but this is not an indication that you are wasting away or entering starvation mode, because after the regular meal time has passed, these thoughts of hunger will usually subside. Try to get your source of carbs from fruits, veggies, and whole grains, and consume a decent portion of protein that fills you up for longer. This is really simple once you get used to eat healthy and understand your body.

2. For quick meals, stock up. Make sure you still have recipes on hand for quick-to-prepare meals like stir-fries, soups, and salads in your refrigerator and cupboards.

3. If you have kids or grandkids don't polish their plates off. Eating leftovers from children is a fast way for parents and grandparents to add weight. When the kids are done with their dinner, place the dishes directly into the sink or dishwasher, so you would not be tempted!

4. Minimize the size of the dinner plate. A great deal of our appetite and pleasure are psychological. We can feel scarcity of

food as we see a large plate that is only half full. However, we can easily fool our mind if the plate is tiny but appears full with the same amount of food; we subconsciously think we have consumed enough.

5. Don't be fooled by the typical "frappucoffee" mixture of milkshake and coffee typical of the most famous fhranchises. That is not equivalent of coffee. Black coffee only contains about 10 calories, but for a regular small cappuccino, a milky coffee can contain anywhere from 100 calories to a whopping 350+ calories for a grand with all the toppings. In the same fashion you shortened your plate size, shrink your cup size and the waistlinewill follow. Don't think about asking for half the milk. Do your own coffee and don't fill the cup to the brim. Less is more when it comes to the joy of savoring the little things.

6. Sandwich is the go-to carb-heavy snack. If you must eat it for time constraints cut the processed carbs losing the top slice of bread and load it up with green salad leaves and few balanced dressing instead.

7. You don't have to make all these life changes at once. You can take it slow, nobody is chasing you, only you. You decide the pace, because you are your best person to assess how your body is doing. Focus on one step at a time.

8. Make sure the portions are right. If you're reducing the number of meals you consume, it stands to reason that the portion sizes should be higher than if you were eating more mini-meals a day.

Use the recipe section as a guide to decide the size of your portions.

9. If you're a mom, or you have baby grandchildren, pick carefully the meals you want to skip. I've attempted fasting with a toddler who couldn't understand why mummy was not eating and one day decided to shove a fistful of tuna pasta into my mouth. Be mindful of the example that you're giving.

RULE 6: GO EASY ON THE BACON

Let's speak about the saturated fats known as LCT, or long-chained fats, which are plentiful in fatty animal products like sausages, pork, fatty beef, and lard. Dairy fats produce around 35% LCT too, however they often contain many other fats that mitigate LCT's harmful impact. Physiologically, LCTs are the best fats in terms of being processed for further use by the liver. They are fat-soluble and, as a result, can survive in fat cells (unlike SCT and MCT); additionally, they do not go rancid. This suggests that LCTs can be retained for longer periods, a trick human bodies have acquired during evolution, and there are a variety of pathways that influence weight gain by making long-chained saturated fats. First and foremost, LCTs decrease insulin sensitivity, which means that more insulin is needed to maintain blood sugar regulation (to unlock the cells, so that blood sugar is absorbed). Insulin is also a hormone that helps the digestion of fats by fat cells. As a result, more insulin makes us fatter!

Since it takes time for insulin sensitivity to deteriorate, a mixture of fats at each meal can have a detrimental effect. Higher insulin and blood sugar levels are caused by eating habits with a large presence of saturated fats, compared to diary regimen with more unsaturated fats. As the saturated fat intake increases, fat burning tends to decline. Today we have far too many overweight children with excessive belly fat whose diets rely on daily high doses of saturated fats rather than watching closely wha they eat. And I find this terrifying.

The Wrong Saturated Fats Are Difficult to Digest

Long-chained saturated fats seem to be slower to metabolise than monounsaturated or polyunsaturated fats throughout the muscles. Olive oil, avocado, rapeseed oil, and fish are rich in monounsaturated and polyunsaturated fats. Long-chained saturated fats are more difficult for the body to burn during exercise, according to reports. This is important for both those who want to lose weight and those who want to improve their stamina and general health to slow down aging.

Products to Avoid if You Want to Burn Fat:

• Bacon

• Pork belly

• Fatty sausages

• Minced pork

• Tallow

• Too many fatty dairy products (cream, butter, cheese)

CHAPTER SIX

Common Intermittent Fasting Myths, Debunked

What I am hopefully you have understood along our journey thorughout this guide is that if you decide to do any form of intermittent fasting, you are not alone. Fasting went from a cult-like knowledge, to trend to lay now on the surface of the public opinion as a common practice.

However, as per all the things that too many people talk about, myths are often created, and the informations provided by the *vulgata* may not be exactly correct. This is why it's vital to discern between fact and fiction. Fasting knowing the truth about any common misconceptions can help us doing it better.

Skepticism revolving around intermittent fasting is due to the many misunderstandings about this dietary regimen. Often the bulk of this derogatory motives is based on close to no research, but on prejudices and stereotypes instead.

Here are 21 myths about intermittent fasting that are worth talking about.

Myth 1: *When you Fast your Metabolism slows down*

When a human loses weight, their metabolism slows down. This is possible, but the effects can be mitigated. When a person deprives themselves of both food energy and stored energy, their metabolism slows down as a defensive mechanism.

The amount of energy expenditure is relatively connected to depriving oneself of calories, which is unavoidable if weight loss is the target. However, if the body can readily access its stored resources, any energy deficiency in it can be counterbalanced, as the body can efficiently use stored fat as an energy source. In theory, individuals with low insulin levels will be able to reach their accumulated fat more quickly, eliminating the need for metabolism to slow down while the body's energy needs are met. When someone fasts, their insulin levels are at their lowest possible levels, indicating that fasting can also be helpful when it comes to metabolism reductions.

Myth 2*: You Shouldn't Drink Water While Fasting*

Religious forms of fasting usually include both the prohibition of food and drink (such as in Ramadan). Possibly unrelated, a variety of arguments that no-water fasts are optimal for health have emerged.

Sadly, because fasting has a diuretic effect, water restriction can lead to hazardous dehydration. That's why when supervising patients undertaking surgical fasts, doctors pay particular attention to fluid consumption. Physicians often pay particular attention to electrolytes, all of which are energetically peed out while fasting, such as sodium and potassium.

So during a fast, drink lots of water and consider potassium and sodium supplements if the fast runs more than 13 or 14 hours.

Myth 3: *Your muscle breakdown while fasting*

Before any substantial amount of muscle is used for energy, one will need to fast for five or six consecutive days. Muscle tissue is constantly broken down and repaired, and by encouraging autophagy, i.e. the clearance of old proteins with the substitution of newer ones, fasting may facilitate this process; less likely to get weakened. This is awesome!

In tandem with resistance exercise, experiments on fasting have actually demonstrated positive effects on the strength and hypertrophy of worked out muscles. In moments of shortage, the body works overtime in order to conserve muscle. Your body switches to body fat (not muscle) for energy requirements when you fast. If we burnt out muscle during a fast, our ancestors would have been unable to hunt!

Myth 4: *Fasting Makes You Overindulge*

You'll be hungry after a fast. This appetite can induce to overeating. Researchers, on the other hand, refute this concern. Many studies on fasting encourage patients to consume as much as they want in a procedure called ad libitum eating. In these studies many subjects eat until full, and are still losing weight.

But of course most intermittent fasting protocols allow to eat less rather than more. In exchange, a well programmed calorie restriction encourages loss of weight without slowing down the metabolism.

Myth 5: *Fasting Is Just Starving Yourself*

Fasting is a voluntary measure to stop eating only for a pre-selected, regulated time span. True hunger is when no food is available, beyond the control of a person, for an undetermined amount of time.

When someone fasts, their circulating insulin levels decrease, suggesting that they are having a stable supply of calories from fat stores and are not 'starving' themselves.

Myth 6: *Fasting Will Deprive You of Essential Nutrients*

Participants of the fasting groups did not exhibit symptoms of malnutrition or nutritional loss in long-term clinical trials. When breaking the fast, the consistency of the foods should be prioritised. Nutritional shortages can be avoided by eliminating packaged, nutrient-poor foods and increasing intake of nutrient-dense, unprocessed foods.

Finally, since fat soluble vitamins are readily available, they have the ability to be released into circulation from fat stores.

Myth 7: *Fasting Just Makes You Hungry All The Time*

According to research, skipping a meal allows people to consume marginally extra at the next meal, but not enough to compensate for the missing meal. Imagine eating 500kcals for breakfast and

500kcals for buffet lunch; missing breakfast the next week and serving the same buffet lunch, eating 700kcals. In this scenario, because they missed breakfast, the person ate more at lunch, but also less overall.

Fasting has been found to decrease appetite hormones and increase satiety hormones, all of which encourage fullness. Some people may feel hungry at first, but once they've developed an intermittent fasting routine, they report feeling less hungry.

Myth 8: Breakfast Is the Most Important Meal Of The Day

The theory behind this is that at the start of your day, breakfast gives you the energy boost you need. Fact is, if you don't eat first thing in the morning, your body will compensate by increasing amounts of adrenaline, growth hormone, and cortisol, which will allow the liver to release glucose, supplying you with the energy you need to start your day. As a consequence, eating when you first wake up isn't essential.

Breakfast is most widely associated with the first meal of the day, in the morning. Once the word is broken down (break-fast), however, it is more 'socially appropriate' to agree that it does not matter when you break your overnight fast.

Myth 9: Fasting Saps Your Energy Food is fuel. Without it, won't your energy levels fall?

Ultimately, yes. Yet your cells tap into an alternative energy supply while you fast intermittently: body fat. There's plenty of it to go around.

And also a slim person has amazing fat reserves to meet energy needs when fasting (e.g., 150 pounds with 10 percent body fat). 15 pounds of fat equals over 60,000 calories of energy if you do the math!

In fact, many people believe that exercising when fasted gives them more energy. It makes sense, given that after a big meal, blood is redirected away from muscles and to digestive organs.

Myth 10: You Can't Focus While Fasting

Remember the last time you were really hungry. Chances are it wasn't your most zen moment. But you can avoid to feel "hangry" if you observe intermittent fasting on a daily basis and train your body to answer to this feeling. Your appetite hormones stabilise as your cells switch to using body fat for nutrition.

Burning body fat also releases ketones, which are small molecules that supply pure, usable energy to the brain. It's been shown that encouraging ketosis increases concentration, attention, and focus in older adults.

Myth 11: Intermittent Fasting Means You 'Just Skip Breakfast'

While most people fast from 8 p.m. to noon the next day, you are free to break your fast whenever you want. You can adjust your hours to suit you, maybe eating from 7am to 3pm, where breakfast is included.

Myth 12: Intermittent Fasting Is A Calorie-restricted Diet

While with intermittent fasting, you may take in fewer calories, this isn't the goal. The biggest distinction between the two is the feeding times. People who follow a calorie-restricted diet eat small, low-calorie meals throughout the day. With fasting you go through exact cycles that cause your body to turn to fat stores for energy - helping you lose weight. In addition, there are usually no calorie limits for your meals in between fasts as long as you consume a balanced diet high in healthy fats and whole grains (while limiting plain refined carbohydrates).

Myth 13: Intermittent Fasting Is For Everyone

While fasting is usually safe and healthy for the majority of people, some cateogries may be required to not make use of it. Kids, pregnant and breastfeeding mothers, and underweight people are part of these categories.

The aforementioned classes need to consume more food, not less. Any possible fasting gains are outweighed by the possibility of nutritional deficiency. Those with elevated blood sugar should show caution as well. Although fasting for this condition may be benefitial, medical care is necessary in order to avoid the eventuality of dangerously low blood sugar (hypoglycemia).

Myth 14: Fasting does not Detox your organism.

One of the strongest components of intermittent fasting is how it decreases the chemical burden and turns your bloodstream into a well-oiled engine.

The mechanism by which your cells remove waste materials, Autophagy, is triggered while fasting. Thanks to autophagy, when you fast you clean out the "junk". This mechanism seems to be necessary for the survival of all of your body's cells and is hotught to be related to a longer lifespan.

Myth 15: *Frequent Meals Can Help You Lose Weight*

Eating more often has little effect on weight loss because it does not improve the metabolism. Indeed, a study on 16 obese people measured the results of consuming 3 and 6 meals a day and observed little change in weight, loss of fat, or appetite.

If anyway, eating more regularly makes you feel better, leading you to eat less calories and less junk food, feel free to stick to it.

Myth 16: *Your Brain Needs A Regular Supply Of Dietary Glucose*

Some say that if you don't consume carbohydrates every few hours, your brain may slow down. This is centered on the assumption that only glucose can be used for food in the brain.

However, through a mechanism called gluconeogenesis, the body can easily generate the glucose it requires.

Your body can produce ketone bodies from dietary fats even during long-term fasting, malnutrition, or incredibly low-carb diets. Ketone will feed all the necessary areas of the brain, decreasing the amount of glucose needed.

Myth 17: Fasting Puts Your Body In Starvation Mode

One common topic against intermittent fasting is that it forces your body into starvation mode, which keeps your metabolism from functioning and prevents you from losing weight.

Although it is possible that long-term weight loss will decrease the amount of calories you burn over time, no matter what type of weight loss you choose, this will eventually happen.

There is no proof that intermittent fasting produces a larger drop in burned calories than other methods to lose weight. In fact, the metabolic rate can be improved by short-term fasting. This is attributed to a dramatic spike in norepinephrine levels in the blood, which increases your metabolism and instructs your fat cells to break down body fat.

Studies suggest that fasting will improve the metabolism by 3.6-14 percent for up to 48 hours. However, the results can reverse if you fast longer, and your metabolism be lowered. One research found that fasting for 22 hours every second day did not lead to a decrease in metabolic rate, but, on average, a 4 percent loss in fat mass.

Myth 18: Intermittent Fasting Is Bad For Your Health

Although you may have heard that intermittent fasting is terrible for your health, evidence suggests that it has a range of health benefits. It has been shown to increase the lifetime of animals by modifying gene expression linked to survival and immunity.

It also has significant metabolic health effects, such as increased exposure to insulin and lowered risk of oxidative stress, inflammation, and heart disease. Increased levels of brain-derived neurotrophic factor (BDNF), a hormone that may defend against stress and various other psychiatric disorders, can also improve brain wellbeing.

Intermittent fasting is one of the highly efficient strategies available as the last resort for burning fats as energy. Since glycogen and blood glucose are reduced in a fasted state, the body is forced to rely on fats for energy. The body is prepared to reach the fasted state when you wake up and fast for around 8 hours.

Myth 19: *Intermittent Fasting Is Bad for Women*

This is a prominent issue that sometimes I hear from women. Experts, on the other hand, have differing opinions. During intermittent fasting, pre-menopausal people may undergo hormonal changes, but this has been verified during very intense fasting. Many women fast for 20 hours a day, and their hormone balance is no concern.

The origin of this misconception on intermittent fasting may be because women are more prone to stress and fasting is a body stressor that leaves some of us unable to cope with it. Some are more adaptable to the pressures involved with intermittent fasting, while some are unable to endure it. So it all relies on you. If you feel good, keep at it, as long as it's beneficial.

On the other hand, if you'd feel some form of disturbance, it is advisable that you start small and gradually increase the periods of your intermittent fasting to allow your body to respond to the changes.

Myth 20: *The Longer Your Fast, The Better*

This isn't right. After 20-24 hours, the effects of fasting start to disappear. However, some findings indicate that fasting for 24 hours, but only once a week, provides greater benefits. After 72-96 hours without food (roughly 3-4 days), starvation mode sets in. So keep it easy and don't overdo it with your fasting time.

The Bottom-line

It's incredible what this easy and efficient eating system can do for the body, brain, and health. As one gets through misinformed intermittent fasting misconceptions, the only unquestionable truth and bottom line is that each of us are made differently, and the only reliable answer is to give heed to your body.

Common Mistakes to Avoid During Intermittent Fasting

1. Being Overly Ambitious with Fasting

I suppose that at our age each of us has learned to feel our bodies: that is the body with we consciously start intermittent fasting. Instead of assuming that you should change your lifetime eating pattern immediately, if sometimes you want food, if it can help you on the longrun, go and calm the hunger. It may take a few weeks for your body to adapt to fasting, but keep pulling those "cheaters" farther apart before you hit a point where you can totally forget about the food and won't want to go back.

2. Not Taking Enough Minerals:

In terms of calories in and calories out, minerals do not effect your metabolism. For cellular functions and for the electrical signals our brain sends in our body, minerals are so essential. The brain does not perform properly if you don't have them, so you can add minerals to your water jug and drink it while you're fasting.

3. Consuming Branched Chain Amino Acids:

An interesting research on the subject: a group of 5 men were selected and their levels of energy substrate, amino acids and insulin were tested during their fasting. On the first day, they took a baseline blood sample and then began fasting. They were given 5 grammes of branched-chain amino acids at the start of their fast. The findings revealed that they had a little insulin spike during the day (note that a little insulin spike in the body makes it difficult to enter into ketosis).

4. Not Exercising:

When fasting, exercising tends to stimulate the metabolism. If you exercise intensely, you can stimulate the sympathetic nervous system, which will induce oxidation and lipolysis (lipid breakdown), which includes the hydrolysis of triglycerides into glycerol and free fatty acids, meaning that fats are being activated.

The human growth hormone rises enormously as you fast and exercise, which consequently facilitates fatty acid oxidation and mobilisation. give it a shot and enjoy the benefits.

Frequently Asked Questions

How can I start Intermittent fasting?

Sleeping. When you sleep you are already fasting. Tray to extend the fasting to lunch with no snacks in between or before bed. Depending on what result you're after it may take some experimenting, Most of the people I know see the first improvements eating in the range 10 am - 6 pm.

Is it a difficult diet to follow?

Intermittent fasting may be daunting at first, however when the body transitions to a different way of eating, the diet becomes more manageable. The basic principle is to be more mindful of what and where you eat.

We encourage physical exercise along with intermittent fasting, eliminating carbohydrates, and picking fruits, vegetables, beans, lentils, whole grains, lean proteins and good fats. The correct exercise routine can be a little difficult to follow, but the rewards of joining them with the fasting can bring to incredible results.

What Is The Most Beneficial Fasting Period?

Fat burning normally starts after 12 hours of fasting and peaks between 16 and 24 hours of fasting.

How Many Days A Week Is Fasting Recommended?

Individuals fast each day for up to 16 hours. Usually, this is achieved by missing breakfast in the morning after eating the day's last meal the day before. As showed in this book there is also a trend of prolonged fasting that allows up to two days a week to go 24 hours without food.

How Much Can I Eat During The Eating Period?

If you want to lose weight, adhere to a calorie intake that helps you to lose one to two pounds every week. On average, you'll need to cut 500 calories a day to shed one pound a week.

What kind of drinks are allowed during fasting?

Water, water, water. When you intend to indulge in fasting, make sure you get plenty of water during the hours when you do not consume solid food. It is also possible to eat vegetables, chicken or bone broth. Soda and caffeine-containing drinks should be avoided.

Are there any benefits of intermittent fasting, including weight loss?

Fasting will help reduce cholesterol, increase glucose regulation, decrease liver fat, and boost blood pressure, in addition to lower body weight. People who make intermittent fasting an habit have strengthened stamina, better muscle control and improved sleep. Eating in line with the circadian cycle (eat during the day, sleep at night) assists in the promotion of deep sleep. Studies have also found that fasting improves the longevity of healthy individuals.

Studies also show that fasting can decrease tumour growth and may help reduce breast cancer recurrences.

Do I cavetto count calories everytime?

No, but if you skip meals before bedtime and go longer stretches without feeding, your calorie consumption will drop, so you should keep them in check, for your well being, especially when you're ì eating foods that are usually lower in calories, for example if you choose a predominantly plant-based diet.

Who Benefits Most From Intermittent Fasting?

Fasting intermittently isn't for everyone. This is a potent tool to have in the toolkit for those who wants to lose weight and are very motivated. In the end, it's about the lifestyle you want and the decisions you make. Ask yourself "What would be the best for me?".

Are There Certain Medical Conditions Where Intermittent Fasting Should Be Avoided?

People with a history of eating disorders such as anorexia and bulimia, and pregnant or breastfeeding women should not try to fast unless they are closely watched by a doctor.

CHAPTER SEVEN

Top Intermittent Fasting Recipes

You'll need substantial go-to meals that will keep you full all day, if you're feeding within a twelve-hour, eight-hour, or four-hour range! If you're considering a high-protein diet for that purpose, you'll find all of the information you need right here, starting from...

SPICY CHOCOLATE KETO FAT BOMBS

Ingredients:

- 1 tablespoon ground cinnamon

- 1/4 teaspoon kosher salt

- 1/2 cup toasted coconut flakes

- 1/4 teaspoon cayenne (to taste)

- 2/3 cup coconut oil

- 2/3 cup smooth peanut butter

- 1/2 cup dark cocoa

- 4 (6 g) packets stevia (or to taste)

Directions

1. In a double boiler set over a pot of simmering water, combine coconut oil, peanut butter, and cocoa powder. Heat, whisking constantly, until the product is molten and smooth.

2. Combine the stevia, cinnamon, and salt in a mixing bowl.

3. Spoon the mixture into a silicone mini muffin tray. (Alternatively, split the mixture among the liners in a mini muffin tin lined with liners.)

4. Top with coconut and cayenne and place in freezer for 30 minutes or until solid.

GRILLED LEMON SALMON

Ingredients

- 2 teaspoons fresh dill

- 1/2 teaspoon pepper

- 1/2 teaspoon salt

- 1/2 teaspoon garlic powder

- 1 1/2 lbs salmon fillets

- 1/4 cup packed brown sugar

- 1 chicken bouillon cube, mixed with

- 3 tablespoons water

- 3 tablespoons oil

- 3 tablespoons soy sauce

- 4 tablespoons finely chopped green onions

- 1 lemon, thinly sliced

- 2 slices onions, seperated into rings

Directions

1. Season salmon with dill, chilli, salt, and garlic powder.

2. Transfer to a small glass pan.

3. Combine the sugar, chicken broth, fat, soy sauce, and green onions in a mixing bowl.

4. Pour the sauce over the salmon.

5. Refrigerate for 1 hour, turning once.

6. Drain the marinade and toss it out.

7. Put lemon and onion on top of grill on medium heat.

8. Cook for 15 minutes, or until fish is cooked.

ROASTED BROCCOLI W LEMON GARLIC & TOASTED PINE NUTS

Ingredients

- 1/2 teaspoon lemon zest, grated

- 1 -2 tablespoon fresh lemon juice

- 2 tablespoons pine nuts, toasted

- 1 lb broccoli floret

- 2 tablespoons olive oil, salt & freshly ground black pepper

- 2 tablespoons unsalted butter

- 1 teaspoon garlic, minced

Directions

1. Preheat the oven to 500 °C.

2. Toss the broccoli with the oil and season with salt and pepper in a big mixing bowl.

3. Arrange the florets on a baking sheet in a single layer and roast for 12 minutes, rotating once, or until only tender.

4. Meanwhile, melt the butter in a shallow saucepan over medium heat.

5. Add the garlic and lemon zest and cook for 1 minute, stirring constantly.

6. Allow to cool slightly before adding the lemon juice.

7. Sprinkle the lemon butter over the broccoli in a serving bowl and toss to cover.

8. Sprinkle the toasted pine nuts on top.

SHREDDED BRUSSELS SPROUTS WITH BACON AND ONIONS

Ingredients

- Two slices bacon

- One small yellow onion, thinly sliced

- 1/4 teaspoon salt (or to taste)

- 3/4 cup water

- 1 teaspoon Dijon mustard

- 1 lb Brussels sprout, trimmed, halved and very thinly sliced

- 1 tablespoon cider vinegar

Directions

1. In a wide skillet, cook bacon until crisp (5–7 minutes) over

medium heat; drain on paper towels, then crumble.

2. Toss the onion and salt into the drippings in the pan and fry, stirring often, until soft and browned (about 3 minutes).

3. Pour in the water and mustard, scraping up any browned bits from the bottom of the pan, then add the Brussels sprouts and fry, stirring often, until tender (4 to 6 minutes).

4. Add the vinegar and crumbled bacon on top.

MAMA'S SUPPER CLUB TILAPIA PARMESAN

Ingredients

- Two lbs tilapia fillets (orange roughy, cod or red snapper can be substituted)

- Two tablespoons lemon juice

- 1/2 cup grated parmesan cheese

- 4 tablespoons butter, room temperature

- Three tablespoons mayonnaise

- Three tablespoons finely chopped green onions

- 1/4 teaspoon seasoning salt (I like Old Bay seasoning here)

- 1/4 teaspoon dried basil, black pepper

- One dash hot pepper sauce

Directions

1. Preheat the oven to 350 °C.

2. Arrange fillets in a single layer in a buttered 13-by-9-inch baking dish or jellyroll tray.

3. Fillets should not be stacked.

4. Drizzle the juice over the end.

5. Add cheese, butter, mayonnaise, onions, and seasonings in a mixing dish.

6. Using a fork, thoroughly combine all ingredients.

7. Bake fish for 10 to 20 minutes in a preheated oven, or until it begins to flake.

8. Spread the cheese mixture on top and bake for 5 minutes, or until golden brown.

9. The length of time it takes to bake the fish depends on its thickness.

10. Keep an eye on the fish and make sure it doesn't overcook.

11. This recipe serves 4 people.

12. Note: You can also cook this fish in a broiler.

13. Broil for 3 or 4 minutes, or until the chicken is almost cooked.

14. Broil for another 2 or 3 minutes, or until cheese is browned.

MEDITERRANEAN CHICKEN BREASTS WITH AVOCADO TAPENADE

Ingredients

- Four boneless skinless chicken breast halves

- One tablespoon grated lemon peel

- Five tablespoons fresh lemon juice, divided

- Two tablespoons olive oil, divided

- One teaspoon olive oil, divided

- One garlic clove, finely chopped

- 1/2 teaspoon salt

- 1/4 teaspoon ground black pepper

- 2 garlic cloves, roasted and mashed

- 1/2 teaspoon sea salt

- 1/4 teaspoon fresh ground pepper

- One medium tomatoes, seeded and finely chopped

- 1/4 cup small green pimento stuffed olive, thinly sliced

- Three tablespoons capers, rinsed

- 2 tablespoons fresh basil leaves, finely sliced

- 1 large Hass avocado, ripe, finely chopped

Directions

1. Combine chicken, lemon peel, 2 tablespoons lemon juice, 2 tablespoons olive oil, garlic, salt, and pepper in a sealable plastic container. Refrigerate for 30 minutes after sealing the container.

2. Combine the remaining 3 tablespoons lemon juice, roasted garlic, 1/2 teaspoon olive oil, sea salt, and freshly ground pepper in a mixing cup. Set aside the onion, green olives, capers, basil, and avocado.

3. Take the chicken out of the package and discard the marinade. Grill for 4 to 5 minutes per side over medium-hot coals, or until optimal degree of doneness is reached.

4. Combine with Avocado Tapenade and serve.

VEGAN FRIED 'FISH' TACOS

Ingredients

- 1 ripe avocado

- 8 small tortillas, vegan mayonnaise, to serve

- 1 red onion, peeled, finely sliced

- 1/4 cup apple cider vinegar

- 1 tablespoon sugar

- 1 teaspoon salt

- 14 ounces' silken tofu

- 2 cups panko breadcrumbs

- 1/2 cup plain flour

- 1/2 teaspoon salt

- 1 teaspoon smoked paprika

- 1/2 teaspoon cayenne pepper

- 1 teaspoon ground cumin

- 1/2 cup non-dairy milk, vegetable oil, for frying

- 1/4 head cabbage, finely shredded

Directions

1. Remove extra moisture from the tofu by patting it with a few bits of kitchen paper. Split the tofu into rough 1-inch pieces with a knife – I like them to be imperfect, rather than cubes, because they look better!

2. Combine the breadcrumbs in a large shallow dish.

3. In a separate large shallow dish, combine the rice, cinnamon, smoked paprika, cayenne, and cumin.

4. Pour the milk into a third shallow wide bowl.

5. Carefully coat the tofu chunks in flour, and milk, then breadcrumbs before placing them on a baking sheet.

6. Pour 1/2 inch of vegetable oil into a deep frying pan. Place over a medium heat and allow the oil to heat up – if a breadcrumb begins to bubble and brown, the oil is ready. Fry chunks of breaded tofu until golden beneath, then turn and finish cooking until golden all over. To drain, place on a baking sheet lined with kitchen paper. Rep for the rest of the tofu.

7. To make the pickled onion, combine the following ingredients in a small bowl.

8. In a small bath, heat the apple cider vinegar, salt, and sugar until steaming. Pour the hot vinegar over the finely sliced red onion in a bowl or pot. Allow it to soften and turn pink for at least 30 minutes.

9. Toss the hot fried tofu with pickled onion, vegan mayo, avocado, and shredded cabbage in warmed tortillas (I warm mine over the stove's lit gas ring).

COBB SALAD WITH BROWN DERBY DRESSING

Ingredients

- 1/2 cup blue cheese, crumbled

- Dressing

- 1/2 head iceberg lettuce

- 1/2 bunch watercress

- 1 bunch chicory lettuce

- 1/2 head romaine lettuce

- 2 medium tomatoes, skinned and seeded

- 1/2 lb smoked turkey breast

- 6 slices crisp bacon

- 1 avocado, sliced in half, seeded and peeled

- 3 hardboiled egg

- 2 tablespoons chives, chopped fine

- 2 tablespoons water

- 1/8 teaspoon sugar

- 3/4 teaspoon kosher salt

- 1/2 teaspoon Worcestershire sauce

- 2 tablespoons balsamic vinegar (or red wine vinegar)

- 1 tablespoon fresh lemon juice

- 1/2 teaspoon fresh ground black pepper

- 1/8 teaspoon Dijon mustard

- 2 tablespoons olive oil

- 2 cloves garlic, minced very fine

Directions

1. Finely chop all of the greens (almost minced).

2. Arrange in a chilled salad bowl in rows.

3. Halve the tomatoes, remove the seeds, and chop finely.

4. Chop the ham, avocado, eggs, and bacon finely.

5. Arrange all of the ingredients in rows around the lettuces, including the blue cheese.

6. Finish with a sprinkling of chives.

7. Arrange the salad in this manner at the table, and toss with the dressing just before serving in chilled salad bowls.

8. Combine with fresh French bread and serve.

1. For the dressing, combine the following ingredients.

9. In a blender, combine all of the ingredients except the olive oil and mix until smooth.

10. Slowly drizzle in the oil while the machine is working, mixing thoroughly.

11. Store in the refrigerator.

VEGGIE PACKED CHEESY CHICKEN SALAD

Ingredients

- 1 cup cooked boneless skinless chicken breast, cubed

- 1/4 cup celery, finely chopped

- 1/4 cup carrot, shaved into ribbons

- 1/2 cup Baby Spinach, roughly chopped

- 2 1/2 tablespoons fat-free mayonnaise

- 2 tablespoons nonfat sour cream

- 1/8 teaspoon dried parsley

- 2 teaspoons Dijon mustard

- 1/4 cup reduced-fat sharp cheddar cheese, shredded

Directions

1.   Mix all ingredients in a bowl so that everything is coated well with the mayonnaise mixture.

2.   Chill in the fridge for at least 30 minutes but you could do it the night before.

3.   Serve.

AVOCADO QUESADILLAS

Ingredients

- Three tablespoons chopped fresh coriander

- 24 inches flour tortillas

- 1/2 teaspoon vegetable oil

- 1 1/3 cups shredded Monterey jack cheese

- 2 vine-ripe tomatoes, seeded and chopped into 1/4 inch pieces

- 1 ripe avocado, peeled, pitted, and chopped into 1/4 inch pieces

- 1 tablespoon chopped red onion

- 2 teaspoons fresh lemon juice

- 1⁄4 teaspoon Tabasco sauce, salt and pepper

- 1⁄4 cup sour cream

Directions

1. Combine the tomatoes, avocado, onion, lemon juice, and Tabasco in a shallow bowl.

2. Season with salt and pepper to taste.

3. Combine sour cream, coriander, salt, and pepper to taste in a separate shallow dish.

4. Spray the tops of the tortillas with oil and place them on a baking sheet.

5. Broil tortillas until pale golden, about 2 to 4 inches from the sun.

6. Sprinkle cheese thinly over tortillas and broil until melted.

7. To make 2 quesadillas, spread avocado mixture equally over 2 tortillas and cover it with 1 of the remaining tortillas, cheese side down.

8. Cut the quesadillas into four wedges on a cutting board.

9. Serve warm with a dollop of sour cream mixture on top of each wedge.

CAULIFLOWER POPCORN - ROASTED CAULIFLOWER

Ingredients

- 1 head cauliflower or 1 head equal amount of pre-cut commercially prepped cauliflower

- 4 tablespoons olive oil

- 1 teaspoon salt, to taste

Directions

1. Preheat oven to 425 degrees.

2. Trim the head of cauliflower, discarding the core and thick stems; cut florets into pieces about the size of ping-pong balls.

3. In a large bowl, combine the olive oil and salt, whisk, then add the cauliflower pieces and toss thoroughly.

4. Line a baking sheet with parchment for easy cleanup (you can skip that, if you don't have any) then spread the cauliflower pieces on the sheet and roast for 1 hour, turning 3 or 4 times, until most of each piece has turned golden brown.

5. (The browner the cauliflower pieces turn, the more caramelization occurs and the sweeter they'll taste).

EASY BLACK BEAN SOUP

Ingredients

- Two cups chicken broth or 2 cups vegetable broth, salt and pepper

- 1 small red onion, chopped fine

- 1/4 cup cilantro, coarsely chopped or finely chopped

- Three tablespoons olive oil

- One medium onion, chopped

- One tablespoon ground cumin

- 2 -3 cloves garlic

- 2 (14 1/2 ounce) cans black beans

Directions

1. In a pan, sauté the onion in olive oil.

2. When the onion is transparent, apply the cumin.

3. Cook for 30 seconds before adding the garlic and continuing to cook for another 30 to 60 seconds.

4. Combine 1 can black beans and 2 cups vegetable broth in a large mixing bowl.

5. Reduce to a low heat and cook, stirring periodically.

6. Switch off the burner.

7. Mix the ingredients in the pot with a hand blender or switch to a blender.

8. Add the second can of beans, along with the mixed ingredients, to the pot and carry to a low simmer.

9. Garnish the soup with bowls of red onion and cilantro.

BEST BAKED POTATO

Ingredients

- 1 large russet potato

- canola oil

- kosher salt

Directions

1. Preheat the oven to 350°F and arrange the racks in the upper and lower thirds.

2. Scrub the potato (or potatoes) vigorously under cool running water with a hard brush.

3. Dry the spud, then poke 8 to 12 deep holes all over it with a regular fork to allow moisture to escape while cooking.

4. Place in a bowl with a thin coating of oil.

5. Season the potato with kosher salt and put it directly on the oven's centre shelf.

6. On the lower rack, place a baking sheet (I used aluminium foil) to trap any drippings.

7. Bake for 1 hour, or until the skin is crisp but the flesh underneath is tender.

8. To serve, make a dotted line with your fork from end to end, then squeeze the ends of the potato together to break it open. It will easily open.

SAUERKRAUT SALAD

Ingredients

- 1/2 teaspoon salt

- 1/2 teaspoon pepper

- 3/4 cup sugar

- 1/3 cup salad oil

- 1/3 cup cider (I use white) or 1/3 cup white vinegar (I use white)

- One (1 lb) can sauerkraut, drained but not rinsed

- One cup celery, chopped fine

- 1/2 cup green pepper, chopped fine

- Two tablespoons onions, chopped fine

Directions

1. Combine diced vegetables and sauerkraut in a mixing bowl.

2. Stir together the sugar, oil, vinegar, salt, and pepper in a small saucepan over low heat before the sugar dissolves.

3. Allow to cool before pouring over the vegetables.

4. Refrigerate for at least one hour.

VEGAN COCONUT KEFIR BANANA MUFFINS

Ingredients

- 2 cups all-purpose flour

- 1 cup granulated sugar

- 1 cup unsweetened dried shredded coconut

- 2 teaspoons baking soda

- 1 teaspoon baking powder

- 1/2 teaspoon salt

- 2 ripe bananas, mashed

    - 1/2 cups pc dairy-free kefir probiotic fermented coconut milk

- 1/4 cup cold-pressed liquid coconut oil

- 1 teaspoon vanilla extract

Directions

1. Preheat the oven to 350 ° F (180 °c). Using cooking oil, spray a 12-count muffin tin. Remove from the equation.

2. In a big mixing bowl, combine flour, sugar, coconut, baking soda, baking powder, and salt. Remove from the equation.

3. In a separate big mixing cup, combine the bananas, kefir, coconut oil, and vanilla. Add to flour mixture and whisk until there are no white streaks left.

4. Divide the batter evenly among the muffin tin wells. Bake for about 30 minutes, or until the tops are golden and a toothpick inserted in the centre comes out clean. Allow 15 minutes for cooling in the muffin pan.

5. Allow muffins to cool fully on a wire rack before transferring to an airtight container or resealable freezer bag and freezing for up to one month. Cover the muffins separately in plastic wrap or foil before sticking them in the pan or bag to protect them from freezer

burn. Muffins can be thawed overnight in the freezer or warmed in the microwave for 20 to 30 seconds straight from frozen.

VEGAN LENTIL BURGERS

Ingredients

- 1/2 teaspoon salt

- 1 tablespoon olive oil

- 1/2 medium onion, diced

- 1 carrot, diced

- 1 teaspoon pepper

- 1 tablespoon soy sauce

- 3/4 cup rolled oats, finely ground

- 3/4 cup breadcrumbs

- 1 cup dry lentils, well rinsed

- 1/2bcups water

Directions

1. Bring lentils to a boil in salted water for 45 minutes. The lentils will be brittle and much of the liquid will have evaporated.

2. In a large skillet, cook the onions and carrot until tender, around 5 minutes.

3. Combine the cooked ingredients, chilli, soy sauce, oats, and bread crumbs in a mixing dish.

4. Shape the mixture into patties when it is still warm; it will make 8-10 burgers.

5. After that, the burgers can be shallow fried for 1-2 minutes on either side or baked for 15 minutes at 200°C.

BERRY CRISP - WEIGHT WATCHERS CORE RECIPE

Ingredients

- 1/2 cups old fashioned oats

- 1/2 cup Splenda sugar substitute

- 8 ounces plain fat-free yogurt

- 1 teaspoon almond extract

- (16 ounce) bag cherries or (16 ounce) bag blueberries

- 1 (7/8 ounce) box jello sugar-free vanilla pudding mix, cook and serve

- One teaspoon cinnamon

- Half teaspoon nutmeg

- 1/4 cup nonfat milk

- Crisp

Directions

1. Spray an 8x8 baking pan with nonstick cooking spray.

2. In a large mixing bowl, combine all of the fruit ingredients and stir well.

3. Combine crisp mix in a separate dish.

4. To make a top crust, spread this mixture over the berry mixture.

5. Bake for 40-45 minutes at 350°F, or until the topping is crunchy.

THE EASIEST PERFECT HARD BOILED EGGS

Ingredients

- 6 large eggs

- water

Directions

1. Place eggs in medium saucepan. Cover with water 1" above the eggs. Place on stovetop over high heat.

2. Get the water to a boil. Remove from heat and cover immediately. Allow for 18-20 minutes of resting time.

3. Pour cool tap water into container, slanting the pot to allow the hot water to escape. Allow eggs to stay in cold water for 1-2 minutes before peeling.

....

WARM ROASTED VEGETABLE FARRO SALAD

Ingredients

- 1 tablespoon olive oil

- 1 cup cracked farro

  - cups almond milk (Almond Breeze)

- 1 teaspoon tbsp olive oil (15 mL)

- 1 tablespoon olive oil

- 1 tablespoon balsamic vinegar

  - sprigs fresh cilantro

- 1/2 teaspoon salt

- 1/2 medium sized eggplant, peel on and large diced

  - tablespoon kosher salt or 1 tablespoon sea salt

- 1 cup cherry tomatoes, washed and left whole

- 1 medium sized zucchini, peel on and large diced

- 6 white button mushrooms, quartered

- 6 garlic cloves, peeled, trimmed and sliced

- 1/2 medium sized red onion, peeled and cut into wedges

- 1/2 teaspoon pepper

Directions

1. Preheat the oven to 400 degrees Fahrenheit (200 degrees Celsius).

2. Salt the eggplant slices generously on both sides in a wide flat pan or baking dish, flip to coat evenly, and set aside for 30 minutes to release excess moisture and bitterness.

3. Place the eggplant in a big mixing bowl after draining and rinsing it. Combine the tomatoes, zucchini, mushrooms, garlic, and onions in a large mixing bowl. Drizzle olive oil over the vegetables and season with salt and pepper, tossing to coat. Transfer the vegetables to a tin foil-lined ovenproof tray. Roast the vegetables for 20 to 25 minutes, or until they are smooth, caramelised, and fork tender. To keep the vegetables from sticking to the grill, stir or rotate them after 10–15 minutes of roasting. Remove the pan from the oven and place it on a cooling rack.

4. In the meantime, clean the farro and wash it in a colander over

the sink. In a 3-quart (3L) saucepot, combine the farro and Almond Breeze. Add a sprinkle of salt and a drizzle of olive oil to taste. To prevent spilling, bring the liquid to a boil over medium-high heat and then reduce to a gentle simmer. Cook the farro for 20 minutes with the lid cocked to one side to allow steam to escape. Remove the pot from the fire but keep it on the stovetop and cover the lid. Steam for an additional 5 minutes in the pot, or until the farro is soft but slightly chewy in the middle. Fluff with a fork after removing the lid.

5. Toss the cooked farro with the vegetables in a big serving dish and gently toss to coat until ready to serve. Combine the olive oil and balsamic vinegar in a mixing bowl and drizzle over the farro salad. Toss to coat and season to taste with salt and pepper. Serve with a squeeze of lemon and new cilantro on top. Serve warm.

TRAIL MIX

Ingredients

- One cup sunflower seeds (raw)

- One cup raisins

- 1/2 cup dried apricot (unsulphured, chopped)

- 1/4 cup flaked coconut (optional)

- 1/4 cup chocolate (optional) or 1/4 cup carob chips (optional)

- cup almonds (raw)

Directions

1. Combine all ingredients in a big container, cover, and shake!

2. Keep the bag airtight. Refrigerate or freeze to preserve the essential fatty acid properties

CAJUN POTATO, PRAWN/SHRIMP AND AVOCADO SALAD

Ingredients

- 300g new potatoes (small baby or chats 10 oz halved)

- tablespoon olive oil

- 250g king prawns (8 oz, cooked and peeled)

- 1 garlic clove (minced)

- spring onions (finely sliced)

- teaspoons cajun seasoning

- 1 avocado (peeled, stoned and diced)

- 1 cup alfalfa sprout

- salt (to boil potatoes)

Directions

1. Cook the potatoes in a large saucepan of lightly salted boiling water for 10 to 15 minutes or until tender, drain well.

2. Heat the oil in a wok or large nonstick frying pan/skillet.

3. Add the prawns, garlic, spring onions and Cajun seasoning and stir fry for 2 to 3 minutes or until the prawns are hot.

4. Stir in the potatoes and cook for a further minute.

5. Transfer to serving dishes and top with the avocado and the alfalfa sprouts and serve.

POACHED EGGS & AVOCADO TOASTS

Ingredients

- Four eggs

- Two ripe avocados

- Two teaspoons lemon juice (or juice of 1 lime)

- Four slices thick bread

- cup cheese (grated, edam, gruyere or whatever you have on hand)

- salt & freshly ground black pepper

- 4 teaspoons butter (for spreading on toast)

Directions

1. Poach eggs according to your preference.

2. Meanwhile, strip the stones from the avocados and cut them in half.

3. Scoop the flesh into a cup with a spoon, then apply the lemon or lime juice, salt, and pepper.

4. Using a fork, mash the potatoes finely.

5. Sprinkle butter on the bread and toast it.

6. Spread the avocado mixture on buttered toast slices and finish with a poached egg.

7. Garnish with grated cheese and serve right away.

. . . .

SWEET POTATO CURRY WITH SPINACH AND CHICKPEAS

Ingredients

- 10 ounces fresh spinach, washed, stemmed and coarsely chopped

- large sweet potatoes, peeled and diced (about 2 lbs)

- 1 (14 1/2 ounce) can chickpeas, rinsed and drained

- 1/2 cup water

- 1 (14 1/2 ounce) can diced tomatoes, can substitute fresh if available

- 1/4 cup chopped fresh cilantro, for garnish

- basmati rice or brown rice, for serving

- 1/2 large sweet onions, chopped or 2 scallions, thinly sliced

- 2 teaspoon canola oil

- tablespoons curry powder

- 1 tablespoon cumin

- 1 teaspoon cinnamon

Directions

1. You can cook the sweet potatoes in whatever way you choose.

2. I peel, pick, and steam mine for about 15 minutes in a veggie steamer.

3. Baking or boiling are both viable options.

4. Heat 1-2 tsp canola or vegetable oil over medium heat as sweet potatoes are cooking.

5. Add the onions and cook for 2-3 minutes, or before they soften.

6. Whisk in the curry powder, cumin, and cinnamon to properly cover the onions in spices.

7. Stir in the tomatoes and their juices, as well as the chickpeas.

8. Pour in 12 cup water and bring to a strong boil for a minute.

9. Next, add a few handfuls of fresh spinach at a time, swirling to cover with the cooking liquid.

10. After all of the spinach has been added to the pan, cover and cook for 3 minutes, or until just wilted.

11. Stir the fried sweet potatoes into the liquid to coat them.

12. Continue to cook for another 3-5 minutes, or until all of the flavours are well blended.

13. Toss with fresh cilantro and serve immediately in a serving bowl.

PEACH BERRY SMOOTHIE

Ingredients

- 1/4 cup coconut milk (adjust for thicker or thinner smoothie)

- 1/2 cup Greek yogurt

- 1/2 teaspoon almond flavoring

- cup frozen peaches

Directions

1. Mix peaches through almond flavoring in a high speed blender.

2. Check thickness and adjust accordingly. Add more milk for thinner and more peaches for thicker.

3. Top with gorgeous toppings like chia seeds, berries and slivered almonds

SWEET POTATO AND BLACK BEAN BURRITO

Ingredients

- 4 teaspoons ground coriander

- 4   1/2 cups cooked black beans (three 15-ounce cans,

drained)

- 2⁄3 cup lightly packed cilantro leaf

- tablespoons fresh lemon juice

- 1 teaspoon salt

- 12 (10 inch) flour tortillas

- fresh salsa

- 5 cups peeled cubed sweet potatoes

- 1⁄2 teaspoon salt

- 2 2 teaspoons other vegetable oil or 2 teaspoons broth

- 3 1⁄2 cups diced onions

- 4 garlic cloves, minced (or pressed)

- tablespoon minced fresh green chili pepper

- 4 teaspoons ground cumin

Directions

1. Preheat the oven to 350 degrees Fahrenheit.

2. In a medium saucepan, combine the sweet potatoes, salt, and enough water to cover them.

3. Cover and bring to a boil, then reduce to a low heat and cook until the vegetables are tender about 10 minutes.

4. Drain the water and set it aside.

5. In a medium skillet or saucepan, warm the oil and add the onions, garlic, and chile while the sweet potatoes are frying.

6. Cover and cook on medium-low heat, stirring regularly, for around 7 minutes, or until the onions are tender.

7. Cook for another 2 to 3 minutes, stirring regularly, after adding the cumin and coriander.

8. Take the pan off the heat and set it aside.

9. Puree the black beans, cilantro, lemon juice, cinnamon, and roasted sweet potatoes in a food processor until smooth (or mash the ingredients in a large bowl by hand).

10. Add the fried onions and spices to the sweet potato mixture in a big mixing cup.

11. Grease a big baking dish lightly.

12. Spoon around 2/3 to 3/4 cup of filling into the middle of each tortilla, roll it up, and put it in the baking bowl, seam side down.

13. Bake for about 30 minutes, or until piping hot, covered tightly with foil.

14. Serve with salsa on top.

PERFECT CAULIFLOWER PIZZA CRUST

Ingredients

- 4bcups raw cauliflower, riced or 1 medium cauliflower head

- egg, beaten

- 1 cup chevre cheese or 1 cup other soft cheese

- 1 teaspoon dried oregano

- pinch salt

Directions

1. Preheat the oven to 400 degrees Fahrenheit.

2. To produce the cauliflower rice, pulse batches of fresh cauliflower florets until a rice-like texture is obtained in a food processor.

3. Put a big pot of water to a boil with around an inch of water in it. Cook for about 4-5 minutes after adding the "rice" and covering it. Drain into a strainer with a fine mesh.

4. Move the rice to a clean, thin dishtowel until it has been strained. SQUEEZE all the extra moisture out of the steamed rice by wrapping it in a dishtowel, twisting it up. It's incredible how much extra liquid can be released, resulting in a clean, dry pizza crust.

5. Combine the strained rice, beating egg, goat cheese, and spices in a big mixing bowl. (Don't be shy of using your mouth! You like it to be thoroughly mixed.) It won't be like any other pizza dough you've made before, but don't worry: it'll hold together!

6. Place the dough on a baking sheet that has been lined with parchment paper. (It must be lined with parchment paper or else it would stick.) Keep the dough about 3/8" thick, and if you like, raise the edges for a "crust" effect.

7. Preheat oven to 400°F and bake for 35-40 minutes. When finished, the crust should be solid and golden brown.

8. Now is the time to add any of your favourite toppings, including sauce, cheese, and all other ingredients you desire. Return the pizza to the oven and bake for another 5-10 minutes, or until the cheese is melted and bubbling.

9. Slice and serve immediately!

SHEET PAN CHICKEN AND BRUSSEL SPROUTS

Ingredients

- 4 skin on chicken thighs

- 1/2 cups Brussels sprouts, halved

- 4 carrots, cut on the bias

- tablespoons olive oil

- 1 teaspoon herbes de provence

Directions

1. Preheat oven to 400° F.

2. Put cut vegetables into a bowl and add 1½ tbsp olive oil, ½ tsp herbs and salt and pepper. Rub all over vegetables.

3. Place veggies on a sheet pan.

4. Add chicken thighs to the same bowl. Drizzle with 1½ tbsp olive oil, ½ tsp herbs and salt and pepper. Rub all over chicken.

5. Place chicken on pan.

6. Roast for about 30-35 minutes or until chicken is done.

7.   If you prefer a crispier vegetable or chicken skin, turn the oven to broil and cook for a minute or two. Watch carefully or it will burn.

BROCCOLI DAL CURRY

Ingredients

- 4 tablespoons butter or 4 tablespoons ghee

- 2 medium onions, chopped

- teaspoon chili powder

- 1/2 teaspoons black pepper

- teaspoons cumin

- 1 teaspoon ground coriander

- teaspoons turmeric

- 1 cup red lentil

- 1 lemon

- cups chicken broth

- medium broccoli, chopped

- 1/2 cup dried coconut (optional)

- 1 tablespoon flour

- 1 teaspoon salt

- 1 cup cashews, coarsely chopped (optional)

Directions

1. In a saucepan, melt the butter and brown the onions.

2. Combine chilli powder, cinnamon, cumin, coriander, and turmeric in a mixing bowl.

3. Cook for 1 minute while stirring.

4. Stir in the lentils, lemon juice, broth, and, if using, the coconut.

5. Bring to a boil, then reduce to a low heat and cook for 45-55 minutes (if mixture is too thick, you may need to add a little hot water).

6. Cook broccoli for 7 minutes in a steamer.

7. Rinse the broccoli and set it aside in cold water.

8. Drain about a third of the liquid from the lentil mixture.

9. Mix in the flour to make a thick paste.

Return to the pan and stir in the broccoli, salt, and nuts, if using.

11. Simmer for 5 minutes on low heat.

12. Combine with Basmati rice and serve.

BAKED MAHI MAHI

Ingredients

- 2 lbsmahimahi (4 fillets)

- lemon, juiced

- 1/4 teaspoon garlic salt

- 1/4 teaspoon ground black pepper

- 1 cup mayonnaise

- 1/4 cup white onion, finely chopped

- breadcrumbs

Directions

1. Preheat the oven to 425 degrees Fahrenheit.

2. Place the fish in a baking dish after rinsing it. Squeeze lemon juice over the fish, then season with salt and pepper.

3. Sprinkle mayonnaise and sliced onions on the cod. Bake for 25 minutes at 425°F with breadcrumbs on top.

4. Spread the mixture out on the prepared baking sheet and bake for 2 hours, or until completely dried. Stirring is not allowed! Remove from the oven and set aside to cool before slicing into chunks. Keep the bottle airtight.

FRENCH VANILLA ALMOND GRANOLA

Ingredients

- 3 1/2 cups old fashioned oats (not quick)

- 1/2 cup sliced almonds

- 1/2 cup water

- 1/2 cup natural cane sugar

- 1/4 teaspoon salt

- 1/4 cup organic canola oil or 1/4 cup grapeseed oil

- tablespoon vanilla extract

Directions

1. Heat oven to 200 degrees F. Line a large, rimmed cookie sheet with parchment paper.

2. In a large bowl mix together the oats and almonds.

3. In a small saucepan over medium heat, stir the sugar and salt into the water. Cook and stir until sugar is dissolved. Remove from heat. Stir in canola oil and vanilla. Pour into the oat and almond mixture and stir until thoroughly combined.

MILLET & QUINOA MEDITERRANEAN SALAD

Ingredients

- 1/2 cup millet

- cup water

- 1/2 cup quinoa (red, white, or black)

- 3/4 cup water

- 1 English cucumber, diced

- 1 tomatoes, ripe, seeds squeezed out, diced

- 1 sweet pepper, seeded, diced

- 1/2 red onion, sliced thin

- 1 garlic clove, pressed

- 200g feta cheese, diced

- 1/4 teaspoon cayenne pepper (more, to taste)

- teaspoons dried dill (sub basil or oregano, if preferred)

- 1/4 cup pine nuts

- 1 lemon, juice of (zest as well, if preferred)

- 1 tablespoon olive oil (optional)

- fresh ground pepper, to taste

Directions

1. Bring 1 cup water and millet to a boil, minimise heat, and simmer for five minutes; remove from heat, cover, and set aside for 10 minutes.

2. Bring quinoa and 3/4 cup water to a boil, then reduce to a low heat and cover and cook for 12-14 minutes, fluffing occasionally.

3. Toss all of the ingredients together and relax. Have fun!

CONCLUSION

Obviously, after we reach menopause, our body and our metabolism shift. One of the most significant differences in women over 50 is a sluggish metabolism, which contributes to weight gain. Fasting might be a safe way to reverse this weight gain and stop it, however. This fasting pattern has been found in research to help control appetite, and people who practise it on a daily basis do not experience the same cravings as others. Intermittent fasting will help you from overeating on a regular basis and attempting to adapt to your slower metabolism.

After you reach 50 your body may also develop certain chronic illnesses including elevated cholesterol and high blood pressure, but the diet we just learnt may come to our help. It has been shown that intermittent fasting decreases both cholesterol and blood pressure, even without a great deal of weight loss. You might be able to get them back down with fasting, even without losing any weight, if you have begun to see the figures rising at the doctor's office each year.

For certain women, intermittent fasting is not a good idea. Make sure to see a specialist before doing any dieting if you are aware you have serious health problems or you're hypoglycemic.

However, for healthy women who naturally accumulate more fat in their bodies and may have difficulty getting rid of these fat reserves, this new dietary pattern has particular advantages. If you are in this category you should definitely give a try and allow yourself to feel better and younger!

To your Health!

J.S.